Heather's Return

From "The We Don't Die" Series

Heather's Return

The Amazing Story of a Child's Communications from Beyond the Grave

by Geri Colozzi Wiitala

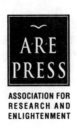

ARE PRESS

ASSOCIATION FOR
RESEARCH AND
ENLIGHTENMENT

A.R.E. Press • Virginia Beach • Virginia

A.R.E. Press
Sixty-Eighth & Atlantic Avenue
P.O. Box 656
Virginia Beach, VA 23451-0656

Library of Congress Cataloging-in-Publication Data
Wiitala, Geri Colozzi, 1943-
   Heather's return / by Geri Colozzi Wiitala.
      p.   cm.
   Includes bibliographical references.
   ISBN 0-87604-351-1
   1. Wiitala, Geri Colozzi, 1943-. 2. Spiritualism—Case stud-
ies. 3. Spiritual biography. 4. Wiitala, Heather Leigh, 1972-
1990. 5. Children—Death—Religious aspects. I. Title.
BF1283.W55A3   1996
133.9'092—dc20
[B]   95-44544

Cover design by Patti McCambridge

Dedication

In Memory of
Heather Leigh Wiitala
October 31, 1972 - September 25, 1990

You were a light in our lives that will burn forever in our hearts. Thank you for blessing our lives with your presence.

Contents

Acknowledgments

During the writing of this book, I was fortunate to receive help and guidance from some special people. Without the gentle encouragement from Dr. Eugene Knott of the University of Rhode Island, the original manuscript may never have taken form. I am deeply grateful to Dr. Knott for helping me to walk through the darkest hours of my life and urging me to journalize my thoughts during this time period.

I am grateful to A.R.E. Press for publishing my story, and I especially thank Ken Skidmore for his valuable contribution as an editor for this book. His kindness, patience, and expertise enabled this story to finally become a book.

I also thank my brother, Dr. John Colozzi, for supplying me with some of my research tools and urging me to continue with my research project. Without some of this historical background, I may not have been secure enough to make some of the changes in my life that I did.

I was very fortunate to have been blessed with some very loving friends and family members. Without them, I don't believe I could have survived this tragedy. Every person named in this story has a special place in my heart and I thank you for being a part of this story. There are other friends and family who are not named but were also supportive and caring; I am blessed to have had you also.

I especially thank my mother, my husband, my daughter Kim, and my sister Fran for always being there. I love you all very much. God bless.

1

The Dream

THE DREAM WAS short. The effect of it began a process that will stay with me forever—a process that previously would have been unthinkable. That is, until Heather died.

Heather died on September 25, 1990, at exactly 7:00 a.m. That was the day that I died also—with her. We buried her three days later on Friday, September 28, 1990. And that night I dreamed of her for the first time since her death. But days before that dream, on the night of September 25, I awoke, with my heart pounding, to something that I still cannot really explain.

There was a figure standing at my bedroom door, staring at me. The bottom of the figure was just a grayish-white form; the head was not easily recognizable. But those blue eyes were intensely staring at me! "Heather?"

It was taller than Heather; it did not look like Heather. But those eyes, those blue eyes. I was terrified! My heart was pounding so hard that I could actually feel it!

I touched my arms to see if I were awake. I was! I closed my eyes. I opened them again, but the form did not move. I assumed that I must be losing my mind in grief, and I closed my eyes again.

I repeated this process over and over again; still, the form did not move. Finally, exhausted, I drifted off to sleep. I assumed that this must have been some sort of hallucination, and I did not tell anyone about it for months.

The days of her death, wake, and funeral are still a blur in my memory: streams of people, oceans of tears, agony beyond comprehension, and endless disbelief and sadness.

Finally, this part of the ordeal was over. Then came the dream. That dream would begin a process that would literally destroy a belief system I had held for close to twenty years and would begin a search that I know will last for at least this lifetime.

In the dream, Heather was lying on the same hospital bed in the same room where she had died. She was lying there—dead. I was sitting alone near the end of her bed, crying. She had a sheet pulled up to her chest and her eyes were closed.

Suddenly, she sat up and looked at me. She said, "I died, didn't I, Mom?" I began to sob and I said to her, "Yes, you did."

She looked at me with those big blue eyes and said, "But, it's OK, Mom, because I'm with you now." I just kept sobbing.

Then she gently asked me to tell her how I felt when she was dying. This was a strange request, and I began to sob uncontrollably as I tried to explain to her how I felt.

I explained that I had kept begging God to let me change places with her. I kept telling God that she was only seventeen and that I was forty-seven and that, if He needed a body, to please take mine instead. Please, God, just let her live!

I told her of the agony and insanity of sitting, just watching your child die when there wasn't a damned thing that you could do about it. And, apparently, God wasn't too willing to consider my request. I told her how helpless I felt in trying to save her and how much I loved her. She just quietly listened to me.

When I finally finished, she took my hand and looked at me very intently with those big blue eyes. Then she said, "I'm so sorry that you had to see me die like that, but I've been resurrected and I am with you, now. It's OK."

Suddenly, I was awake. I was sobbing, but I was awake. That dream has never left me, even to this day. I know that it was a dream, but it was so real—and so contradictory to what my religious system had taught me.

I tried to share this with my older daughter, Kim. But she said to me, "Mom, you know that can't be possible. She is sleeping until the final judgment."

I said, "I know." But doubts were beginning to grow with each passing day. Things began to happen. And I began to see a very different picture starting to emerge. Very slowly, very gradually, the process began.

2

The Process

*"Ask, and you will receive; seek, and you will find; knock,
and the door will be opened to you."*   Matthew 7:7

A T T H E T I M E of Heather's illness and death, I was in a
highly structured, well-organized, Bible-based religion. To
question their doctrines was heresy. And, to be honest, I
never thought of questioning my religious doctrines. Why
should I?

All Christian religions base their teachings on the Bible.
The Bible is held in high esteem throughout the world.
The Bible is used to swear in witnesses and to make U.S.
presidents. And, in this organization, to question its Bible
teachings was equivalent to questioning God and the organization itself (which were sort of synonymous to me at that

time). That was unthinkable. Who was I to question all that wisdom?

Yet, we humans are unique creatures. Our subconscious or our unconscious mind finds ways to fool our conscious mind. At the time of Heather's death, I did not seek to question God or my Bible teachings. Believe me, if at any time one needs a belief system to truly work, it's at the time of a dearly beloved one's death. It would be equivalent to carrying around a parachute on your back and believing it will open when you jump from 10,000 feet. The problem only comes into focus when it doesn't open at that crucial moment. That's equivalent to what happened to me.

For about twenty years, I had been an avid Bible student. I had read and studied the Bible from cover to cover approximately five times. I had read, studied, and taught portions of scripture hundreds of times. My religious system did teach the Bible thoroughly (according to its theory), and I did learn scripture very well. In addition, I hold two master's degrees. I had taught and counseled in a public school system for over twenty years. I consider myself to be reasonably intelligent. So, what was the problem I seemed to be having here? Why was my belief system not holding up at this time?

I tried to get logical with myself. Since my dream experience was contradictory to my beliefs and my elders weren't very happy with my questions, I tried to resolve the issue in my own way.

I reasoned that since I believed in the Bible, yet also believed in my dream, I would read through the Bible specifically looking for dreams and for the possibility that God gives us messages through dreams. In that way, I was not trying to contradict the Bible, God, or the organization (again, these were all synonymous to me at the time).

Well, what a surprise I received! I found that throughout the whole Bible, God constantly communicated to humans through dreams. Further, He promised that even during the last days He would give visions and dreams. This was truly a revelation to me.

It wasn't because I was unaware that dreams were in the Bible. The revelation was more in the way I now became focused. I became very aware of the important role that dreams played in the Bible. But, even more important, I became aware of the role that dreams have in our lives today.

Dreams were no longer just ancient history to study in a Bible class. I somehow became focused on how important this channel of communication between God and humankind was in our very day. I realized the beauty of the gift of dreams that God has given to us and how close it keeps us to Him now. This aspect was truly a revelation to me at that time.

Since I was meeting opposition from my religion's elders, I began to keep my research quiet. My doubts were becoming magnified each day. My fear was also heightened.

To leave this organization meant the loss of all friends and family who remained in the system. I would be condemned to death with no hope of a resurrection. But, worst of all, I would never be allowed to see my beloved Heather again, according to the doctrines of this religion. I just couldn't risk that. I had lost so much when I lost Heather. What could I do now?

I decided to quietly investigate what other Bible-based religions had to say. I first began by watching every religious show that came on cable television. Week after week, I watched every one I could find.

I also began to secretly read scholarly books on religion and the Bible. My search was so intense that it took me weeks to finally figure out what some may conclude to be quite simple. It was as if "I couldn't see the forest for the trees." Perhaps, only if you have been involved in a mind-control system could you relate to this.

At first, the only thing that I could see was how much alike they all were. I would watch the speakers on TV so intently that I would sometimes get a headache. I would observe certain things to be the same for all the speakers.

First, they all looked sincere as they began. Second, they all waved or held the Bible and said it was God's word. Third, they would ask you to go and get your own Bible version and follow along with them. In this way, you would see that what the speaker was saying was really in the Bible (and not just something the speaker was making up).

Fourth, they would tell you what scripture to look up (for example, John 1:1) and read along with them. Fifth, they would actually read the scripture aloud as you followed in your own version. Sixth, they would continue with their discourse, citing more scriptures along the way, until the conclusion.

And do you know what? They were all right. Not once in all the weeks that I did this were any of them wrong. I used six different versions of the Bible; I was able to find every single text that was selected. And I could honestly see the same meaning in the version I chose as compared to the version that the speaker was using.

I was really stumped now. I had listened to close to fifty lectures by many different religious persuasions, and whatever the speaker lectured on, sure enough, those scriptures were there and were appropriately fitting. I wondered, then, what made these groups different? It's important to realize that we were not allowed to attend other religious meetings or even to listen to them on television. So, I truly was perplexed.

Slowly, however, the answer emerged. When it did, it was so obvious that I couldn't believe that I had not seen it immediately.

What I came to discover was this: Although all the speakers looked (and probably were) sincere—and although, when you looked in your own Bible version, the scripture really was where it should be—the answer was actually found right *after* the speaker read the Bible quote. As soon as the speaker finished reading the text, he would say something like "and this means such and such." He would then proceed to go on with the rest of the discourse.

It took me a long time to hear these quick "and this means" and to realize that the speaker was actually interpreting the scripture according to his/her own theology and incorporating this interpretation into the rest of the discourse to arrive at the desired conclusion. It was no wonder that almost every discourse I listened to made sense according to the speaker's personal interpretation. Following this methodology, anyone could make a case for anything and still be able to prove it.

This was getting crazy. Was the difference only in the way someone interpreted a scripture? That's kind of scary when you give this thought serious consideration. Yet, slowly but surely, this point grew to be more and more obvious to me. I read and reread portions of highly acclaimed and scholarly works. I read and reread portions of scripture in various Bible versions. And, I began to see that many different pictures could be painted with the same colors, just as many different (and sometimes radically opposing) religions could be born out of that same Bible. I was devastated.

I had been taught and had believed that there was only one way to read that Bible. And, based on that fact, there was really only one true religion. I remembered having the Bible verse, "one faith, one Lord, one baptism," drilled into my head. My religion taught that this meant only one true religion. And, you guessed it! Theirs was the only true one. How was it possible that suddenly all of these religions made sense when they used and read from that same Bible?

Millions of people have died or been murdered in the name of religion. So surely, my dilemma was not so farfetched.

Nonetheless, I was truly horrified! I felt as if the rug were being pulled out from under me. What would I now do?

3

The Dilemma

"My child, my child . . . O that I might have died instead of you."   *II Samuel 18:33*

THE DEATH OF a child is considered to be the most traumatic death that a person can experience. According to some bereavement experts, a mother suffers most when a child dies. Because she generally bonds to her child from conception on, part of the mother dies with her child. From my own personal experience, it's not just a case of thinking that this is true; it's a case of knowing that this is true—a knowing that I wish that I did not possess.

This was the frame of mind that I was in when this horrific religious dilemma began to rear its ugly head. Yet, from a psychological point of view, it is interesting to observe my first reaction when my mind began to sense that a very serious problem was brewing.

Shortly after I had started my "secret" Bible reading and TV watching, I did what I consider to be an amazingly contradictory thing: I signed up for more hours in my organization's ministry. This increased my ministry up to sixty hours per month.

In this way, I would be doing more evangelizing and conducting more Bible studies to help indoctrinate people. It's important to mention this because this move could have prevented any further spiritual enlightenment. But, in actuality, it would turn out to be a blessing in disguise.

Although I don't recall ever having heard of the word *synchronicity* before, I would eventually come to understand that this process of "meaningful coincidence" had been working in my life the day that Heather died. I am further convinced that this process is always in effect in our lives, but that many of us are sometimes unaware of it.

The Dictionary of Spiritual Thought describes this Jungian term as: "The coincidences of life that reveal the greater, unitive pattern existing outside our normal awareness or perception; what appears as separate actions developing and moving toward a single point of connection; often considered divine timing, sometimes recognized, sometimes not."

This definition of *synchronicity* helped me to understand my coincidental experiences. More important, it has helped me to appreciate a dimension beyond what we humans normally see.

I also came to learn that my move to become deeper entrenched in my religious structure is more common than one would realize. It is motivated by fear and a need for protection.

As I said, this unusual move would take an interesting route. Shortly after I began to increase my hours in the ministry, I came in contact with a Baptist minister. I had been studying with one of his congregation members for over a year now. He informed me that he had been aware of this and was not very concerned because he had felt that her faith was very strong.

Now, however, she had become ill and was terminal with cancer. She was getting weaker, and he did not think that it was fair for her to have doubt raised about her faith at such a crucial time.

I understood and agreed with him. I tried to explain that my purpose was not to weaken her faith but to share Bible truths with her. He told me that he felt that I was misled and was trying to mislead her. He pointed out that, since our organization had made many false prophecies, they were to be viewed according to the Bible text of Deuteronomy 18:20-22: "But the prophet, which shall presume to speak a word in my name, which I have not commanded him to speak, or that shall speak in the name of other gods, even that prophet shall die. And if thou say in thine heart, How shall we know the word which the Lord hath not spoken? When a prophet speaketh in the name of the Lord, if the thing follow not, nor come to pass, that is the thing which the Lord hath not spoken, but the prophet hath spoken it presumptuously: thou shalt not be afraid of him."

I immediately denied that we had ever made a false prophecy. I did this because I had honestly never seen any of them. He told me that if I were sincere, I would check out this information. He offered to bring me a copy of one of the false prophecies. Naturally, I accepted this challenge.

This challenge made it necessary for me to eventually research the history of the organization, history that I was unaware of and very shocked to uncover. My mind actually resisted this information at first and I was almost unable to digest the material that I was uncovering. Fear seemed to encapsulate me.

Several years would pass before I would appreciate and understand why he had urged me to do this research and how crucial it really was for me to know. From a counseling standpoint, this information was necessary for me to grow and heal.

I would also come to remember the bittersweet issue that had divided my friend Evelyn and me. She believed in an immediate resurrection of spirit, and I believed in a bodily resurrection (if you were lucky) at the final end. It turned out that Evelyn was right. I never did get to tell her this because she died a few months after her minister had showed me one of the false prophecies and before I was able to complete my research.

Without her, her minister, and my increased ministry, I might not have come across this essential piece of information. Coincidence? I doubt it. I was truly seeing synchronicity in action in my life. What seemed like a foolish move from a human point of view would actually turn out to be a blessing from a spiritual point of view. Roots were truly starting to take hold within me.

Only my husband, Walt, and my daughter, Kim, knew that I was living a double life. I would work the ministry and attend all of the meetings; but, every other waking moment, I was diligently involved in my research. I was secretly trying to determine how one would know which (if any) of the religious interpretations was correct. Was there really only one true religion on the face of the earth during this time period? If so, which one was it?

At this point, I was intensely angry. I was, also, severely grieving. I felt as if everything were falling down around me and I didn't have a clue as to how to put it back together again. The perfect religious picture I once had had just seemed to disintegrate before my very eyes. I seemed to be looking at a blank canvas.

I very angrily questioned why God would allow my faith to be shaken at a time when I needed it the most. But this mean little voice inside of me said, "Are you kidding? God let you sit and watch your child die right before your eyes!

So, why does it surprise you that He would let your faith be shaken, too?"

Surely, my own death would have been much easier to accept. I began to understand what the word *hell* truly meant. I was in the deepest and darkest part of it right now. It wasn't hot. It wasn't reserved for later. It was now.

As I look back to this time, I realize that I was severely grieving two major losses in my life simultaneously—the loss of my daughter Heather and the loss of my religion. I had become involved in my religious organization about one year after Heather was born. Coincidentally, the death of Heather and the final death of my belief system would also occur within that year.

What's really tragic about the situation is that I had joined this organization as a protection from the impending Armageddon, slated for 1975 (and then changed to any day immediately after that). I had feared greatly for my children. According to their theology, any person who was not baptized into their organization (or a minor child of a baptized member) would be permanently destroyed in this end-of-the-world scenario referred to as Armageddon.

I had stayed in the organization because I had believed that Armageddon would occur at any day (even though those days turned out to be almost twenty years). I had so feared my children's deaths, as well as my own death. Yet, the fear never saved Heather. Heather died anyway and not from Armageddon. I had truly existed (not lived) for almost twenty years in deep fear. Believe me, fear is not a protection. It is a prison.

In my grief, I would cry out to this unseen God and beg Him to tell me what He wanted from me. Why was I alive and wishing I were dead? Why did my child have to die when I so desperately needed her to be alive? Since I didn't have the ability to create the universe and understand the "all" of God, I really didn't think it was very fair of Him to require this of me. To make matters even worse, the nightmare of Heather's final struggle for her life had now reawakened and was in full bloom in my head. I had left the stage of denial or shock (as some grief experts explain) and I was now painfully conscious of the horror and permanence of Heather's death. I couldn't seem to get the answers I so desperately needed from any place. I found this to be so cruel.

Believe me, I had never been fond of the idea of either Heather or myself dying. But, I knew beyond the shadow of a doubt, that if Heather died and I lived, it would be worse for me than if I had actually died instead. I knew that I would never be the same if she died.

My mind was now waking up and vividly reliving those final hours in Heather's struggle for her life. I was remembering what I had so desperately tried to forget. I screamed inside! My body was in agony! I was remembering how I had really wanted to run and not have to look at her dying. At the same time, I knew that I could not leave her side. She needed me more than ever. I had to stay and help her to fight for her life.

I remembered how I had wanted to cut the sky open and attack something, but I didn't know what. I had wanted to grab my child back from "it" and pull her inside of me as when I had carried her in pregnancy. I wanted to hide her from the "thing" that was pulling her out of this realm!

But, in the end, the "thing" won and I lost; and, believe me, I lost it all! There is no greater agony than to sit and watch your child die before your very eyes. The horror of this made me wonder about what kind of a God could allow this to happen.

I remembered that I was supposed to have been her "cheerleader" in urging her to fight for her life and not to give up. I remembered how I had refused to listen to her when she kept telling me that she was dying.

Angrily, she had said to me, "Mom, I'm dying and this is so unfair! I fought so hard to win this battle (with cancer) and now I'm going to die to this infection. This is so unfair!"

I was half-crazy over hearing these words. I kept saying to her, "No, you're not; no, you're not!" I couldn't bear the thought of her dying!

Suddenly I heard her say, "Then why is it getting black?" I panicked! I looked at the monitor. I saw the numbers go into the teens and I gasped at her nurse, "Donna!" I pointed to the monitor as Heather's voice faintly said, "I'm going. Bye."

A screaming noise came from some machine that made a flat line. Doctors and nurses came running into her room. Was I screaming or was it that machine?

I yelled loudly, "Heather, fight! Don't give up—fight!"

I remember doctors pulling me away. I was taken to another room. And my daughter's last words to me would stay with me forever; so would my own stupid last word, "Fight." No person had ever fought harder to live than Heather. What was I saying?

Oh, yes, they managed to bring her back for nineteen more hours on a respirator, and they worked around the clock as I watched. I kept telling her how much I loved her and that she was going to make it. They told me that she couldn't hear me. Yet, a few times she shook her head "no" very vigorously, and I knew that she had heard what I had said.

She knew she was dying. I think that I, too, began to believe this for the first time. As she slipped away, I just sat there slipping away with her. The war was over. The "thing" I hated had finally won.

Heather officially died at 7:00 a.m. on September 25, 1990. Me, too! Why did I have to stay here on planet Earth (or was it really planet hell?). I didn't know why but, for some reason or another, I was here and she was gone. Where? I had no idea.

As I said, so much was going on in my brain simultaneously. My belief system was really bottoming out at the same time that my memory of Heather's death and last hours were being reborn. The reason for my being here suddenly had no purpose. My life seemed so pointless. I felt dead. When any feelings of life dared to enter my body, they were either intense anger or intense grief; and I mean intense! I don't recall too many in-between stages at this time.

I would run into Heather's room to constantly check for something. I wasn't sure what I was checking on, but I think I was hoping that I would find her there after all. But she wasn't there. I would stare at her pictures and frantically cry out, "Heather, where are you?"

As this "civil war" raged inside of me, I began to wonder if anything (like a God) was really out there. If so, which if any religion was the right one?

It was also at this time that I began to understand what the word *zombie* truly must mean. It was I, a shell of a person who used to exist. I even figured out what the expression "a fate worse than death" probably referred to. It meant watching your child die and you live!

As this dilemma reached peak proportions within me, the "God, why?" question was driving home a point of stark reality within me. I finally realized (or at least I had the courage to admit it) that I hated this concept of God!

4

Realization

"My God, My God, Why have you forsaken me?"

Matthew 27:46

I T H I T M E hard when I realized or at least admitted that I hated this concept of God. I had worked a ministry for this God for almost twenty years now. I had talked to Him, prayed to Him, begged Him, bargained with Him, worshiped Him, and, now, I hated Him. I hated this version of God (which later I came to realize was a human-made concept). I had always thought that I had believed in Him and had loved Him. However, I came to realize that I had actually feared this God so much that it would have been virtually impossible for me to ever have really loved Him.

So, I finally told Him so. I shouted at Him, I screamed at

Him, and I hated Him! As I relived the nightmare of Heather's death, I came to realize that the "thing" that was grabbing for Heather and the "it" that I had referred to in my journal was, in actuality, my concept of God. The refusal to name the "it" or "thing" in my journal was the horrendous fear of admitting this hatred aloud.

Sure, there were hints and doubts and suspicious quick flare-ups over this God issue, but now it was like a wall in front of me. I hated this concept of God, and I was glad that He now knew it. I felt as if I had been fighting the wind and wearily I finally just gave up. I concluded one of two things here: either there was no God or, if there was a God, He was powerful, but He was not very loving as I had once assumed Him to be.

With this new realization, many feelings began flooding into my body. The most conspicuous feeling that came forward vividly was fear. With this fear, however, also came a choice. As this "hate God" or "no God" realization smacked me in the face, I was struck with what this horrific fear very obviously implied. If there really was no God, then, when I died, I would never see my beloved Heather again.

That hit me like a ton of bricks. I was crying so hard that I could barely contain myself any longer. O my God, what a sick joke that would turn out to be, I thought.

I went from wishing that I were already dead to a state of almost paralysis. Total fear, total horror, and total sadness surrounded me. Slowly a question formed in my mind. I remember thinking, If there really is no God and if I really will never see Heather again, how will I choose to live the rest of my life?

Without consciously realizing it at that moment, I had acknowledged that I had some choice here. And, from the depths of my being, from thoughts to verbalizing, I was choosing to live my life with love. I heard my own voice say aloud, "Even if there is nothing after this, I will still try to live my life loving my fellow human beings." It seemed as though I instinctively desired to do this no matter what the outcome was to be.

Time would reveal what a very powerful and essential part this would have in my healing. I was realizing that, God or no God, reward or no reward, I still had a choice. What would I choose to do with the rest of my life? And, without initially realizing it, I had chosen to love.

Time has gone by since I made that choice, and I realize what a profound awakening this really was for me. For the first time in my life, I realized that I wasn't afraid of God anymore. A deep sense of peace seemed to enter inside of me at this moment. I didn't understand what was happening right then. It would take time for me to appreciate the value of this awakening.

At this point, my research and reading materials had been limited to Bibles and scholarly reviews of scripture and the history of religions. I had also been able to get some old original literature that my religious organization had published many years ago. All of this, however, was to be only the beginning of my research.

I noticed that I had been thinking with some sort of what I will call "dictionary mentality." My mind would see a scripture and, without any effort, the organization's interpretation would enter into my head. No other interpretation seemed to have been possible.

This seemed to suddenly change. I began to notice that I had developed a strange new way of thinking about scripture. I would visualize the scripture in my mind, but, when I attempted to process the interpretation, it seemed as if a screen would open in my mind and many possible definitions (or interpretations) would enter. It was still like using a dictionary, except now there was more than just the one possible meaning that I had been accustomed to seeing. And, with these expanded definitions, came the sense that none of them was right or wrong. They were all acceptable, depending on the context of the material being used.

I found this to be intriguing. I had no idea what was happening. I felt my mind was shifting gears, and I was functioning with a different gear ratio. I actually seemed to be knowing or understanding at a different level than before. I couldn't seem to put my finger on how I knew, I just seemed to know.

As these facts about religion began to make me question so much, I thought that perhaps my logic needed to be checked. I decided to seek bereavement counseling because I noticed that time was not easing my grieving; if anything, it seemed to be intensifying. I began to wonder if perhaps my grieving wasn't affecting my mind and maybe (just maybe) my logic on the organization's concept of God was wrong. Maybe the process I had chosen for evaluation was incorrect. Since I, myself, am a counselor, I knew that this was a necessary consideration.

I called to make an appointment with a counselor who had been our university's department chairman of counseling until his retirement several years ago. He had been a professor of mine during the time I was working on my M.S. degree in counseling and we had developed a close friendship. I wanted to consult with him now on some of the issues that were confronting me. However, I discovered that he was still in Florida and would not be back in the state for a couple of months. Since I could not reach him, I decided to put this mission on hold for a while.

Coincidentally, later that day a flyer from the Candlelighters Organization arrived in my mail. This flyer announced that a lecture on grieving would be given by another former professor of mine. I had a deep respect for this man. I knew that he, too, had lost a child from a struggle with cancer. However, since this lecture would be given right next door to the hospital where Heather had died, I just could not bring myself to go there even though I desired to hear him speak.

So, I did something that I had never done before in my

life. I called the professor to tell him why I could not attend his lecture. Why I did this, I still do not know. This was a free public lecture with no R.S.V.P. required. Yet, I felt compelled to call him and explain why I could not attend.

That call began a series of events that would prove to be crucial in my healing. It would also enable me to gather more information for this new concept that I was now forming about God and spirituality, a concept that I didn't even realize I was forming at the time. I thought that my spiritual canvas had become blank; I soon would notice the dots that would begin to appear.

As I placed that call, I wondered if he would be in his office and what I would say to him. He was in, and, as soon as he began to talk, I began to cry. I told him that I needed to talk to someone who could help me to deal with my grief. I felt that the grief was getting worse with time instead of easing up as I thought it should. I wanted to know how he was able to function again in society after the loss of his child, since I felt that I could not and would not be able to do this again. Worse yet, I didn't seem to want to anyway. I never mentioned religion at that time. I'm not sure why, but I just didn't.

I was so relieved when he told me that he would be glad to work with me. A ray of hope seemed to appear. As he started to set up the first appointment, he asked me several questions. First, he asked me what kind of cancer Heather had. I knew this question was not needed to set up the appointment but was more of a question in passing.

When I answered him, I simply told him that Heather had bone cancer, since very few people are aware of the rare kind of cancer that she had. I noticed that he had paused a moment. He asked me somewhat hesitantly, "Was it Ewing's sarcoma?"

I was surprised that he was so well versed on the names of the various cancers. Perhaps this was helpful to him in his profession. Nonetheless, I answered a startled, "Yes!"

Again he seemed quiet. Then, he asked me if the cancer had been in one of her ribs. I was totally stunned now. I could not imagine how he could possibly know that, since it is usually found in a limb. I answered with another startled, "Yes," followed by the question, "How did you know that?"

Again he was silent for a moment. Then he asked me if the cancer had been the actual cause of her death. With that I began to sob uncontrollably. I finally blurted out, "No, she beat the cancer and died to an infection!" He very gently murmured, "I'm so sorry."

As I gained my composure, I heard him ask, "Did you ever read *Fireflies?*" I actually wanted to shout at him at this point and say, "Of course not! I am deeply embedded in this insane religious dilemma and I only read religious material!" Naturally, I didn't say that. I just told him that I had never heard of it. I guess I was wondering why he was asking me that.

He then told me that he would bring the book with him when we met the following week. He explained to me that there were some striking similarities between me and the author of that book. He also thought that it would help me to get in touch with my grief. He had no idea that he was about to hand me the key to unlock Pandora's box.

It would be weeks before I would learn that although he had purchased the book over a year and a half ago, he had just read it two weeks before I called him. That was where he had learned the name "Ewing's sarcoma." He himself found this an uncanny coincidence. He, too, would learn that this was just the beginning.

He gave me *Fireflies* on that first visit, and I read it immediately. It was the first book, other than religious books (or school books), that I had read in many years. I not only read that book, I felt that book. I knew the protocol, and I felt as if I were floating through that hospital while the author told his story. My heart went out to him.

The book also contains a few mystical experiences. This was my first exposure to this concept in almost twenty years. I came away from this book considering the possibility of something after death existing, but having no idea as to what it really was. I was far too disillusioned with the "God Thing" to try to analyze the what and how of it all. It was, however, food for thought. Little did I realize it then, but a new seed was truly being planted in my mind. Another dot was beginning to appear on my canvas. Where these dots were going, I did not yet know.

I was sort of fearful about this "mystical stuff." Could it be a trick of a so-called "devil"? Yet, I can honestly say that I was more curious than I was fearful at this point. I now had a desire to know. This desire was about to be fueled.

5

The Calla-Lily Incident

"I will pour out my Spirit . . . sons and daughters . . . will prophesy . . . will see visions, will dream dreams." Acts 2:17

A S I L O O K back, my TV watching, my readings, and my research were all very necessary steps for me in my growth and my healing. Now, with counseling being added, I was beginning to feel more secure about not knowing all the answers to the "God Issue." My counselor, Gene, was truly a gift. I was very comfortable with him, and it wasn't long before I began to tell him all about my secret research and my double life.

I asked him if the process I had used to evaluate religion was logical. He told me that it was indeed. He also had a problem with the doctrines of this organization. He began to loan me other books to help me to expand my very narrow perspective of God and life. God must have been in on all of this because I had just finished reading *Fireflies* when the strangest and most involved incident happened in our home.

It was now May and I was reliving Heather's prom experience. She had been crowned queen of the senior prom the year before on May 18, 1990. I looked at her prom pictures and, wig and all, she was truly beautiful. Her classmates will probably never know how much it meant to her to be chosen by them to be their queen. I am deeply indebted to them for that.

She had been one year into her battle with cancer and she had missed a lot of school. She had lost weight, lost ribs, and she had lost her hair. To a seventeen-year-old girl, the hair loss is traumatic. Yet, Heather would get up, put on her makeup, put on her wig, get dressed, and she would look really beautiful. Her prom night was no exception.

She had designed her own gown. She intended to be a fashion designer one day. Designing and making her own gown proved to be good therapy for her. She did a great job. She selected the most beautiful and unique bouquet that I had ever seen at a high-school prom. She had chosen three large calla lilies to be held together with the same royal blue color as her gown. The florist did an excellent job in designing this bouquet. It was lovely.

She looked so beautiful that night. She was on the queen's court, and this made her feel very honored and happy. This happiness was a boost to her immune system and you could visibly see the radiance about her. Being chosen as the queen was the frosting on the cake for her. She was ecstatic. When I hear the expression "in her glory," I would have to say that this was truly Heather's night of glory while living on the earth.

I cried as I looked at her pictures and remembered that special night one year before. I cried as I thought of what could have been if it weren't for the infection at the end. I was sad and I was bitter at the same time.

Then, from out of nowhere, a thought crossed my mind. I would order the same kind of bouquet that she had carried for her prom, and I would bring the bouquet to her grave on the anniversary date of her prom. I thought that she would probably be glad that I had remembered such a happy day in her life. It had meant so much to her.

I ordered the bouquet a week ahead of time since these flowers are not always in stock. I asked that they be delivered late on Friday, May 17, so that I could bring them to the cemetery early on the morning of May 18.

A day after I placed the order for the bouquet, we received a phone call from Canada. Brian, a very dear friend and one of Heather's pallbearers, wanted to make a quick trip down to visit for the weekend. We were delighted. We hadn't seen Brian since the funeral, and we were looking forward to his visit.

Brian arrived on the afternoon of May 17 and brought with him his fiancé, Judy, whom we had never met before. Shortly after they arrived, the bouquet was delivered. We explained its purpose to Brian and Judy. We put the bouquet into a large cooler next to Heather's bedroom door. Walt and I had decided to stay in Heather's room for the weekend and have Brian and Judy stay in our room upstairs. In that way, I could go to the cemetery early in the morning and not disturb anyone who was still sleeping.

Since Brian was well known by many of our friends, people stopped by the house to visit with him. Everyone saw the bouquet and agreed that it was a good idea and that Heather would be happy that we had remembered her prom day.

After everyone left that evening, Brian and Judy retired upstairs to rest from their nine-hour journey. Walt also decided to retire for the evening. I stayed up for a while cleaning the kitchen and getting things ready for morning. It was close to midnight when I retired for the evening. The house was quiet as everyone was already sleeping.

I'm a light sleeper and usually awake early. It was about 6:00 a.m. and I was getting up to make some coffee. Suddenly, Walt woke up and said to me, "Heather was here last night!" This was an odd way of putting it, and I assumed that he meant that he had a dream about her.

I said to him, "Do you mean you had a dream of her? What was it about?" He looked at me very seriously and half-whispered, "No, I said that she was here last night!"

This sounded crazy. Walt was an atheist at that time, and it was totally out of character for him to make a statement like this. So, I asked him again what he was really trying to tell me. He became annoyed with me and said, "I tell you, Heather was actually here last night!" I asked him, "How do you know that?"

He explained to me that he had been in a deep sleep, but that a feeling of intense warmth (not heat) had awakened him. He said that he was lying there for a few minutes trying to figure out what was producing the sensation of warmth in him. Since Walt is a building contractor and had designed and built our house, he knew that our heating system (which is radiant heat) was located in the ceiling. But the warmth seemed to be coming from beside him and near the headboard of the bed. He also knew that the heating system had been turned off, since it was a mild night.

He further explained that, just as he seemed to have determined the location of this heat source and was wondering what could be the cause of it, something began to move near him.

He saw something that he described as "a mist" or "a cloud" begin to move slowly beside him. This cloud (or mist) felt as if it passed right through him and then began moving into the wall next to where he was sleeping. It disappeared into the wall at a point right next to a large 45" x 45" contemporary design that Heather had created in art class. He explained that he couldn't see its face, but he just knew it was she.

I asked him how he could know that for sure. He said, "I'm telling you, I just know; it felt so warm, so peaceful, and so close; and I can't explain how I know it was she, I just know." His eyes filled with tears as he dropped back down on his pillow.

This conversation in itself was unbelievable. Walt was the atheist. I was the one into religion. He never wanted a part of religion, and he believed in nothing. He thought that Heather was dead—forever.

Although I, at this time, also believed that she was totally dead, I at least believed a future resurrection was possible at the end times. I just sat there for a minute quite stunned by this conversation. I knew that something had truly happened to Walt, but I honestly just didn't know if such a thing were really possible.

I finally got up to go and make the coffee. As I began walking, I noticed a picture lying face up on the floor near the sliding glass door. One glance and I knew what that picture had to be.

It was a Polaroid® shot of Heather standing alone in front of the sliding glass door and holding her calla-lily bouquet. It had been the first picture that we had taken of her on the night of her prom. I had wanted an instant picture of her that night and there was only one Polaroid® shot left in the camera. The rest of the pictures had been taken with a regular camera and were much larger. So I knew what the picture was before I even picked it up.

I remembered that I had taped the picture to a glass vase on her prom night. That picture had been on the vase (containing silk roses) for a year now. This vase was on top of her bureau with many other pictures and items.

I glanced over to the bureau where the vase and other pictures were, and I noticed that a 5" x 7" framed picture of her was lying face down on the bureau. The vase was still standing, but the Polaroid® picture was obviously no longer taped to it. The framed picture had been situated directly in front of this vase. It was now lying face down.

Words can never adequately describe how I felt at that moment. I had no idea what had happened or how it had happened. Considering the snapshot, I looked back and forth from the bureau to the sliding door (a distance of at least six feet). I said, "O my God, how did this picture get over to here?"

There were several large plants between the bureau and the middle of the eight-foot sliding door. There was also a one-inch lip along the top of the bureau. There were no windows open. I was trying hard to understand how the picture could get over to where it was, even if the tape had let go and the picture had fallen off the vase. However, I also could not figure out what caused the heavy gold frame to be just lying face down. Why had nothing else been moved or disturbed on the bureau?

Heather's bureau top was very cluttered and had remained exactly the same way that I had arranged it shortly after her death. The only thing different at this moment was that the Polaroid® picture was off the vase and the framed picture was face down. This was absurd.

I am a light sleeper and all of this movement would have taken place about two feet from where I had been sleeping. I would have been awakened by the noise of the heavy frame if the 5" x 7" had fallen down on the bureau; even so, how did the Polaroid® get untaped from the vase and end up halfway across the room? What caused the movement?

Walt had sat up to observe what I was apparently describing aloud. His eyes were as big as saucers, and his face was almost pale white. I was close to being hysterical at this point.

As I stood there rambling on and on, Walt just murmured, "See, I told you. Heather was here last night." He dropped back onto his pillow and began to cry. I just stood rooted to my spot, holding the picture of my beautiful Heather. I was shaking.

Apparently, Brian had heard the pitch of our voices and thought that something was wrong. He came downstairs to see what all the commotion was about. As he entered the room, I began to ramble on about the pictures and about Walt's encounter.

Brian just stood there solemnly listening to us. He is a retired Royal Canadian Mounted Police (RCMP) and had worked as a detective for the Canadian government. I would consider him to be pretty solidly based in reality, so I asked him if it were possible for the tape on the picture to lose its grip and fall that far away from the bureau.

Brian observed the layout. Then he quietly said, "Let's be realistic here; there is no way that this just could have *happened.*"

He pointed out the lip around the bureau's edge and the fact that there were no windows open. He also observed that there was nothing wrong with the picture frame and that the frame was very sturdy. He concluded that there was no logical explanation for why the snapshot ended up in the middle of the room and the picture frame was lying face down. Since he observed the rest of the bureau to be undisturbed, he felt that it was a very selective movement. Further, he didn't have a clue as to what could have possibly happened to Walt. He just knew that it was out of character for Walt to express something of this nature.

I was now sensing that Brian seemed to be getting more emotionally involved in this discussion than what I would have expected him to be. He then looked at us solemnly and said, "I have something to tell you that is really going to blow your mind now."

He proceeded to tell us that during the night Judy had awakened to see something standing at the foot of their bed. Since the door to the bedroom had been closed, she couldn't figure out how someone could be there or who it could be. Since she really didn't know us, she wondered if we might have entered to get something we needed, but she really didn't think we would do that. She then wondered how the person got in the room and why the person would just stand at the foot of the bed.

She tried to recognize the person but could only determine a form standing still at the foot of the bed. She then thought that Brian was trying to play a joke on her. She lay still and waited for the form to move. It didn't.

She began to panic and thought that a thief had entered somehow. She slid her leg quietly under the covers to nudge Brian and wake him up. She could feel him sleeping beside her and she nudged him harder.

Brian awoke startled. Judy began to tell him about the form at the foot of the bed, but the form seemed to just disappear. Brian jumped out of bed.

He put the light on. There were no windows open and the door was still shut. The bedroom appeared to be undisturbed as did their luggage. So they went back to bed puzzled by this encounter. They were going to tell us about it the next morning. Little did they realize what must have been going on downstairs.

Our conversation had become so loud now that Judy awoke and hurried downstairs. As she entered the room, we all seemed to say at once, "You won't believe what happened last night." Judy grew pale and half-whispered, "What? Were we really robbed last night?" She then tried to explain to us what caused her to wake up in the first place.

She told me that she woke up because she felt movement beside her. She explained to me that she could almost hear the movement, but could not see anything until the form stood at the foot of her bed. As she listened to the rest of our story, she told us that the hair on her arms stood up. She was truly amazed by the drama that had taken place during the night.

We spent most of the day discussing this with any visitor

who happened to come by. It was interesting to note that all of us came from different religious backgrounds. Brian is an Anglican, but does not consider himself to be overly religious. Judy told us that she had been reared as an Irish Catholic, but had not been to church in years. Walt had been an atheist (but was rapidly changing his mind). And I (at the time) was still a Jehovah's Witness and would consider this all impossible if not actually demonic. Believe me, I wasn't too fond of this phenomenon happening at this moment in my life. I definitely did not solicit this; if anything, I was still sort of frightened by it all.

I would eventually come to view this in a very different light. I would come to see the gift. I would also come to realize that the religious persuasion of a person really had nothing to do with this phenomenon. It was on a much higher level, the spiritual level, that this phenomenon was concerned with. Time would make this clearer.

We took Heather's bouquet to the cemetery that day. I think that we all expected something spectacular to happen. It didn't. The usual happened instead. The tears rolled down our faces and the dense sadness could be felt. We still kept thinking of what could have been and what we felt should have been.

We returned back home and again shared our experiences with our visitors. Elwood, a major in the state police, is another person very solidly based in reality. Yet he, his wife, Cynthia, and his daughter, Heather (whom our Heather was named after), agreed that there was no logical explanation here. They, too, believed it was an encounter beyond the normal range of human experiences. They, however, viewed it as a gift. (I wasn't quite there yet.)

As we shared this experience with other friends (some also do police work), no logical explanation could be found. They know us quite well; they knew something different had truly happened on that special prom anniversary night. It's just that none of them seemed to know what it all really meant.

The one thing we all do know is that many of our lives have been deeply affected and altered by this experience. Personally, it gave me tremendous courage to continue my search—a search that would eventually enable me to get out of a cult that I had been locked in for almost twenty years.

As I mentioned before, only Walt, Kim, and most recently Gene knew about my secret research and my double life. I was now beginning to share this with my friends and family for the first time. I did not share this with any members of my religious sect, except my dear friend Carol. I was still not sure of what was really happening, and I could tell that Carol was frightened by this new person who seemed to be emerging in my body. Thank God she stuck by me and we are still very dear friends to this day.

My friends (outside the religion), family, and colleagues were only too happy to accommodate this new me. Some of them began to give me other reading material (material I would have never before taken). A new circle of knowledge began to emerge. We all started sharing our books and our thoughts on religion, God, and spirituality. Growth soon became apparent in all of us.

As we reflect back to this experience now, we realize that this experience seemed to have served as a catalyst for our personal internal searches. We have become so much more spiritually aware and so much more reluctant to pass judgment.

I also found myself remembering the form that was standing near my bedroom door the night that Heather died. Was it really Heather? Although I still can't be positive, I feel that it was her rather than just an angel. More important, I believe that Heather exists. So do the rest of my friends.

As I reflect back to this prom anniversary, I think that it's interesting to note that Brian called us to initiate the visit. Interestingly, he called within twenty-four hours after I had ordered the bouquet. He was not aware of Heather's prom date or its importance to her.

He told us that he had not had any intention of coming down at that time. He actually always came in mid-summer, as he preferred the warmer weather so that he could go out on Walt's boat. He told me that he wasn't sure what made him change his mind. He just seemed to have the thought come to him, and he acted on that thought. I would learn the power of thoughts in time.

I can see the synchronicity here. I sometimes wonder if, after I placed the flower order, the thought was given to Brian to come and bring Judy (a person we didn't know) as verification for the event that was to take place. Perhaps God was setting things in motion for an appearance by Heather. God (above anyone else) knew what a scared "doubting Thomas" I was. Was He supplying me with evidence so that I would believe it was more than an overactive imagination? I'm sure that He's pleased that I've improved somewhat in this area.

God knew, also, that there could not have been any better teaching mechanism for us at this time than our beloved Heather. If anything were to impact on us now and cause us to grow, it would definitely be she.

Whatever the complete explanation is, I can't be positive. I do believe that it was Heather's spirit that appeared to Walt and Judy; and I do believe it was Heather who appeared to me on the night that she died. As her dream reassured me, she is with me now.

I became aware after all this that my fear was truly being diminished. I was now ready for more.

6

A Different Focus

"I was found by those who did not seek me; I revealed my-
self to those who did not ask for me."   *Romans 10:20*

MY RESEARCH, THE counseling, and what I refer to
as the "calla-lily incident" had brought me to the realization
that something was truly out there even if I didn't understand it. With this realization was a growing sense of it being
OK that I didn't have all the answers any more and perhaps
I never would while I lived on this earth.

In fact, it seemed as if I had fewer answers now than when
I was deeply entrenched in my religious structure. Yet, at
the same time, I felt that I had begun to acquire faith and
peace for the first time in my life. Faith in what? I wasn't
quite sure, but I still felt OK about it.

I reflected back to those first few visits with Gene in my counseling sessions. Those were the times of the "hate God" or "no God" rantings. At that time, I was very serious (perhaps fearfully serious) about voicing this nasty thought aloud. I remember when I said it, I almost held my breath and looked around, wondering if I were going to be struck dead immediately for this wicked thought.

But, come to think of it, I really didn't care then either. Death, at that point, would have been a welcome means of getting me out of my misery. I now had to smile as I remembered explaining to Gene all of these hateful, guilty feelings.

I remembered Gene quietly (but seriously) saying to me, "It's OK, Geri, I think God is big enough to handle your anger. I really don't think that He's going to hold it against you." I smile when I think about this conversation now. I've yet to remind Gene.

As I reflect back to this period in my life, I can't help but think about the story of Jonah. It's worth rereading the fourth chapter of Jonah just to see how angry he was with God. It's more interesting to see how God humored Jonah for a bit and then drove home the point in this parable. This story helps me to keep things in perspective and to lighten up when I'm feeling negative.

Although *Fireflies* could be considered the catalyst for my desire to read material other than that of a religious nature, my personal experiences coupled with the loss of fear were actually essential in my quest to learn.

I was now curious as to how the medical/psychological profession viewed life after death. I began to read the works of Dr. Kübler-Ross, Dr. Moody, Dr. Weiss, Dr. Siegel, Dr. Morse, Dr. Chopra, Dr. Borysenko, Dr. Peck, Dr. Komp, Dr. Ring, Dr. Ritchie, Dr. Dyer, and nurses and other professionals who were working with the dying and their families or with hospice.

Life magazine, coincidentally, came out with an article on "Life after Death" at about this time. I began to become aware of the fact that there was a lot of information out there.

Where had I been all of this time? It was as if I had existed in a vacuum. Was all this information just coming out now for my benefit? I hardly think so. The answer was more in the way that I was now being focused, and—to top it all off—I hadn't requested nor desired this new focus.

I came across a tape by Dr. Dyer entitled "Transformation" and had to laugh as he quoted the famous Taoist expression, "When the student is ready, the teacher arrives." Well, universe, I was ready. Let the lessons begin. I was overwhelmed and amazed that there was so much of this kind of material out there.

I felt like a kid in a candy store. I had been faithful to my religious structure and had pretty much read only their literature and believed only their interpretation. This was a whole new world opening up to me, and these people were not "quacks." These were people who were highly respected in the medical/psychological community.

I remembered my early days of secretly watching all the religious shows that I could find on television. Now, it seemed as if shows on TV were often featuring the mind/body connection and the concept of life after death.

So again, as I read books dealing with this new focus, I would watch every TV show that I could find on this new area. How could I have missed all of this? It had to have always been there. Why had I never noticed it before? Was I blind?

I learned that there were close to thirteen million people who claimed to have had near-death experiences, which were called NDEs. I had never heard of this before. I inhaled this new information at an amazingly rapid rate. Their stories were fascinating. The fact that children as well as adults (and even atheists) had encountered this phenomenon made it all the more believable for me.

It was also at this time that I came across the work of

Edgar Cayce, America's most famous psychic, who is commonly referred to as "the sleeping prophet." Today his "readings" or psychic discourses are researched and studied internationally. He has also been featured in many television programs and has been the subject of hundreds of books.

Coincidentally, a catalogue was accidentally placed in our mailbox. This catalogue featured books about Cayce. At that time, I didn't pay much attention to where the catalogue came from. Instead, it was the name Edgar Cayce that struck me. Where had I heard that name before?

This greatly interested me because I remembered having heard about him some twenty years before from several of my colleagues at the school where I was then teaching. I remembered that I had just begun studying the Bible with the Jehovah's Witnesses at the same time that these colleagues were reading books about Edgar Cayce. John, one of my colleagues, knew someone who had been given a psychic reading by Cayce. The accuracy of that reading was phenomenal. We had great discussions on Cayce, religion, and the Bible.

I remembered how I tried to share this with my Bible study conductor. He highly discouraged me from reading Cayce's work and even called him "demon-possessed." I became frightened because I knew that Armageddon would be any day then. So I clung closer to their organization and stayed clear of the Cayce material. A sad mistake, indeed, but I now realize that I wasn't ready for this part yet.

I have truly come to believe that everything happens for a reason, whether we understand it at the time or not. And I have come to realize the truth of "When the student is ready, the teacher arrives." I was not ready then.

I not only read through the catalogue that day, I immediately placed an order for several Cayce books. I ordered *Edgar Cayce's Story of Karma, Edgar Cayce's Story of Attitudes and Emotions,* and *Edgar Cayce's Story of the Origin and Destiny of Man.*

As soon as my order arrived, I began to read about this man Cayce. I was deeply affected. Why had I not chosen to learn about him twenty years before?

Many people are attracted to the work of Edgar Cayce because they have an interest in holistic medicine or psychic phenomenon. Since many consider Cayce the father of holistic medicine, it is understandable why they would be drawn to his work. I, however, was viewing him as a pioneer in the ecumenical movement and was, therefore, attracted to the spiritual/religious aspect of his work, probably because of the religious dilemma I was in at the time.

As I lamented over this lost time, a friend of ours, Mike, happened to notice that I was reading about Cayce. He was thrilled because he had just become a member of the Association for Research and Enlightenment (A.R.E.), the organization founded by Edgar Cayce to investigate his psychic readings.

He gave me a copy of one of their book catalogues. What was happening here? I scanned the catalogue and immediately ordered *Discovering Your Soul's Purpose* and *God's Other Door.*

When these arrived, I read them immediately. Mike and I had great discussions on Cayce and his works. He showed me the literature from A.R.E. and I decided to become a member.

To read the Cayce material was fascinating for me. I had been an avid Bible student over these last twenty years and I really did know my Bible quite well by now. Perhaps that is one of the positives in my experience with religion. To see Cayce discuss scripture enabled me to view the Bible in a whole new light. I found him so much more loving and freeing in his approach to the Bible and scripture. It was amazing to me how this man could have known what he seemed to intuitively know.

Cayce was a Christian and read the Bible from cover to cover every year of his life. Yet his work actually *stressed* the importance of comparative study among belief systems throughout the world. His focus was always on the oneness of all life, tolerance for all people, and compassion and understanding for all religions.

What I found most interesting, however, was that Cayce would not generally have been considered a "learned man" by our educational standards. Yet, here he was, urging comparative study of all religious systems. By studying all the major belief systems a person would be able to discern the oneness of them all. I began to realize what a vital key Cayce was urging humankind to use. This would be a unifying concept for all of us. The outward structures that seem to cause division and strife on the earth could feasibly be replaced by the oneness of spirit that exists in all humanity. How could this man possibly know this?

My mind raced back to my early days of secretly watching religious TV shows. I remembered how at first I could only see how much alike they all were. I had to strain my brain to find the differences. Was God, through Cayce, trying to tell me something again?

These varying interpretations seem to be what makes them different, yet they also make them divided instead of united. I remembered Jesus' words, "You will know the truth and the truth will set you free." (John 8:32) The concept I was now learning was truly freeing to me indeed.

The Bible's reference to one faith that I had been taught to believe meant only one true religion now took on a very different meaning for me. In reality, we really are all one. Even Jesus alluded to this when He explained that He and the Father were one and that all the followers would become one. God is Love; to love is what makes us all become one.

I am deeply indebted to Cayce and to all of the other people who have given me a piece to this universal puzzle. Each of these writers has given me a unique piece and I am grateful for that.

The blank spiritual canvas I once thought I had now seemed to have dots here and there. There was no definite picture yet, but something was obviously being created.

I noticed that I was less angry and less fearful now. I realized that I didn't need to have all the answers any more. Everyone's path is different. I was so relieved.

Suddenly, the Bible passage, "Faith is the substance of things hoped for, the evidence of things not seen" (Hebrews 11:1), seemed to stand out in my mind. I realized that I was actually developing faith (and not just facts) for the first time in my life.

7

The New York Adventure

"Now about spiritual gifts ... there are different kinds of gifts ... All these are the work of one and the same Spirit, and he gives them to each one, just as he determines."

I Corinthians 12:1, 4, 11

APPROXIMATELY A WEEK or so after the calla-lily incident, Kim and I came upon another aspect of this unusual phenomenon. It was nearing the first memorial of Kim's father's death. Joe, my first husband, had died one year before on May 29, 1990. That was also the day that Heather was accidentally chemically burned on her wrist, causing the wound that four months later would become infected and result in her death.

Kim had recently made contact with Robyn (who had been engaged to Kim's father at the time of Kim's wedding some ten years before). Although Joe and Robyn had eventually parted ways, Kim had always kept a special place in her heart for Robyn. Since Kim had not heard from Robyn, she wondered if Robyn knew that Joe had died.

Kim had been trying to contact Robyn through her previous address at her mother's house. Robyn's mother had forwarded the letter and Robyn had finally made contact with Kim.

Robyn shared an experience with Kim. She told Kim that Joe was alive on the "other side" (as Robyn called it) and that she had made contact with him through a famous psychic named George Anderson. Robyn gave Kim a copy of the book *We Don't Die* and urged Kim and me to try to contact George in regard to Heather.

Since I had only just begun to do research in the medical/psychological field, I found this concept totally bizarre. I did, however, make a mental note to contact Robyn secretly so as not to involve Kim. Since we were both still technically enrolled in our religious organization, both of us knew that this would be considered demonic and grounds for disfellowshiping at that point. My desire was to protect Kim from this happening.

As soon as Kim left me that day, I called Robyn's mother to get Robyn's number. As I chatted with her, she told me that she had accompanied Robyn to see George Anderson and had made contact with her deceased husband, Sal. She told me that George had allowed them to tape the hour session and that Kim and I would be welcome to hear the tape.

I called Robyn to get the information on George. She also urged me to listen to her tape so that I could get an idea as to how a session was conducted. She felt that he was knowledgeable and legitimate. She told me that he had told her many things that were true and that he would not have had any way of knowing any of these things. She urged me to call for an appointment, but told me that he was very difficult to contact. It had taken her almost a year to get one.

I asked her to keep this conversation confidential and she

promised me that she would. I thanked her for the information and hung up the phone. Since I was late for an appointment, I quickly got into my car and left.

I had driven about one mile from my house when I suddenly noticed something quite unique. As I passed by a local restaurant, I couldn't help but notice the license plate of one of the cars. It read, "BROPHY." That was Kim's father's last name.

Obviously it was not his car. It belonged to a distant relative of his who ran a local business. But what really stood out in my mind at that time (since I hadn't yet learned the word *synchronicity*) was that I had never seen that plate before (nor have I since) and I had just hung up the phone from talking to Robyn only five minutes before.

To reinforce this train of thought, the song from the movie *Ghost* came on the radio. I remember feeling very odd and thinking of how coincidental this all seemed to be. The phone call, the license plate, and the song seemed somehow to fit together at that moment in time.

I found myself reflecting on how I had not seen Robyn in ten years; yet today I had spoken to her just five minutes before seeing Joe's last name on a license plate. I also found it odd that Kim would finally make contact with Robyn at this particular time in our lives.

I vowed to contact George, but to not tell Kim. Walt and I discussed this with several of our friends. Elwood and Cynthia decided to accompany us to New York if we could get an appointment.

To get an appointment with George in those days involved calling a certain number on the first Tuesday of the month between 6:00 to 8:00 p.m. That was it. There was no other time or way that we knew of to get through to him. And, if the line were busy for the whole two hours, we would have to wait another month to call again. Robyn warned me that it could be very frustrating to try to get an appointment, but she felt it was well worth it and urged me to persevere.

I was lucky that the first Tuesday of June was within a few days, as I am not a very patient person. I excitedly sat at my phone from 6:00 to 8:00 p.m. with my finger constantly punching the redial button for those two hours. I cried when 8:15 arrived and only the busy signal could be heard. I had actually started dialing fifteen minutes before the hour with the chance that I could get through early. But no such luck; the constant busy signal was truly agonizing to hear.

I phoned Robyn to tell her the news. She urged me to try again in July and invited Kim and me to hear her tape of George. I told her not to tell Kim that I had called George and was planning to try again next month. She agreed to keep it a secret. We set a date for lunch for the following week.

Kim and I met with Robyn and her mother and listened to the tape of George. We were both truly amazed to hear the dialogue and have Robyn and her mother confirm the accuracy of the accounts and the names given in the reading. My desire to contact George was tremendously enhanced by listening to the tape and having the information verified. We also became aware of his second book, *We Are Not Forgotten*, and bought a copy. I vowed to call again.

When the first Tuesday in July arrived, I was anxiously at my telephone station repeating the June behavior. Approximately one hour into this redialing mode, a voice answered. I almost fell off my chair as I stammered through the appointment set-up. We were given the date of July 22, 1991, and instructions on how to confirm this appointment.

Although I requested a private reading then, I was told that there were only group reading openings, and I would have to keep trying if I wanted a private reading. I took the group reading and was informed that the group would number close to twenty people.

I called Robyn and told her of our success. I again cautioned her not to tell Kim and she agreed. I told her that Walt and I and Cynthia and Elwood were going by limo to

New York and that I would tape the reading for her to hear. She was pleased.

I could hardly wait for the day to arrive. About a week before the appointment, Kim came to visit. Suddenly she said to me, "I'm going with you."

I asked her what she was talking about and she told me that she had suspected that I had gotten an appointment with George and had tricked Robyn into confirming this. She said that Robyn had then given her the number and told her that she would probably not be able to get through to George.

Surprise! Not only was Kim able to get through to George, I was shocked to learn that she was able to get through to him immediately.

I had not wanted to involve Kim because she had married into a family that was heavily entrenched in our religion, and I knew that this could cause tremendous hardships for her and her children. If I had managed to keep what I was doing a secret, I reasoned that she would be better off not knowing. But God must have chosen otherwise because she was able to get through in spite of the odds.

Five of us made that trip to New York on July 22, 1991. Our appointment was for a 7:00 p.m. reading. Since there were twenty people in the room, it was almost 11:00 p.m. before our turn arrived. Although we were extremely anxious to have our reading so that we could leave (it was a three-hour journey home), there was actually an advantage to our being read so late.

We were able to listen and watch George interact with all of the other people in the group until it was our turn. Many of these people were bereaved parents from the Compassionate Friends group of Long Island. We listened intently as George named events, circumstances, and names for each of these sets of parents. Judging by the number of "yeses" heard, the tears shed, and the appreciative nodding of heads, we could see that these people were verifying the information that George was passing on to them.

It's important to point out here that I was very skeptical of this type of an experience at that time in my life. Something inside of me wanted to know and believe, but the "fundamentalist" side of me was still very overpowering then.

Perhaps that is why we were given our reading at the end of the evening rather than right at the beginning. It took me well over a year to even begin to put this particular event into perspective. Listening to this on tape (in conjunction with my memory of the other people's responses) finally enabled me to accept this type of a gift. To be honest, at the time it was happening, I was still trying to find loopholes and trying to analyze how he could possibly do this. Where was he getting this information?

At approximately 11:00 p.m., George felt the pull to come over to Elwood and Cynthia. I was glad that they were before us because I could watch how they responded to the information that George gave them as they taped their reading.

George told them events, circumstances, and names of people of which at that moment Walt and I were not even aware. We have been very close friends for over twenty-five years, and yet there were things told to them of which we had no prior knowledge. I could hear and see Elwood and Cynthia verifying the information George was now giving to them. Even more so, I could tell by their body language that they were very moved by the information in this reading. "Why am I being so skeptical?" I thought. Later on the way home, they did confirm and explain the information about which we had previously not known.

When Walt, Kim, and I were approached, I tried to sit as expressionless as possible so as not to give George any clues. The first person to come through to us was my father. He told me things about my mother's health that were correct.

The next person to come through was probably Joe (Kim's father), but I missed the cue. I assumed he was talking about my Uncle Nick who had just passed over the month before. Later, after listening to my tape several times, I realized that he was probably discerning Joe.

The dialogue is so rapidly given (depending on the people trying to come through) that if vital cues are missed, George will assume that the entity does not have a connection to you or that he is not interpreting the symbols correctly for you to understand. He will then pass over the information and focus on the other information coming through. His book *Our Children Forever* would give the reader a good idea as to how our reading was conducted.

Since I was so new to all of this at that time, I missed vital cues that could have given us even more information. As I review our tape now, I wish that I had been more alert then; yet we still received very vital and accurate information.

Obviously, the most important pieces of information began to come when he suddenly asked me, "Do you take the name of Heather?" I felt as though my heart were being squeezed, and I had trouble holding my composure at the mention of her name. He had already described enough of Heather's personality and intimate circumstances of her death for us to realize that it was she whom he was dealing with. But when he actually said her name, it really hit me!

He named one other name and this truly stunned me also. Heather's best friend through her school years was Christina. They had doubled dated the night of the prom. Christina had stayed with me one night at the hospital when Heather was in crisis. She had slept in our home in Heather's bed. A card for Heather from Christina that says "Best Friends" still hangs on Heather's mirror.

Probably the deepest connection for me was that she had been the only person to ask me if she could put a letter into Heather's casket. Of course, I told her she could. No one ever read that letter, and I have no idea as to its content. So, when George said, "Tell Christina that you've heard from me," I was truly amazed.

Four years would pass before we could actually share this tape with Christina. She was amazed that this could be possible. She agreed that if I had tried to share this with her before, she would not have been able to accept it. She, too, needed time. As she listened to the tape, she said to me, "Geri, he is using phrases and words that Heather would actually say to me at times. He sounds just like he is actually talking to her."

We eventually shared this with Kim's grandmother, Miriam (Joe's mother). I wondered how she would feel about all this. She surprised me when she told us that she believed it because shortly after her own father died, she had had a strange experience herself. She told us that, as she lay in bed grieving for her dad, a hand covered her own hand very gently, and she felt that it was her father comforting her. Kim and I found this reassuring.

Another key point for me was when George asked me if I was bothered by the fact that I wasn't there at the minute Heather had died. This rather startled me because I had truly lamented over this fact. Why had I walked out of the room just a few minutes before 7:00 a.m. on that day?

George also told us that Heather's cancer was located in the chest area and that the cancer had not been the cause of her death. He started to add onto this information at one point and asked us if she had breast cancer (a natural assumption), but before we could even answer him, he told us that she had sternly corrected him and told him to repeat only what she had said (which was the chest area). He was correct, since Heather's cancer was located in her rib cage.

He remarked to us that she was a "feisty little one," but a very loving and very beautiful spirit. He told me that she was very forgiving and that she had adjusted fine on the other side. He told me that she was working with other young people who had just passed over. Obviously, I have no way of verifying this particular part, but I would like to believe that this is also true.

George then told me something that was very significant to me. He told me that Heather said that both of the dogs were with her. First of all, I didn't know that animals could go over to the other side. Secondly, I tried to correct him and told him that we had only one dog. He retorted that she had said two dogs and that he wasn't going to argue with her about it.

Suddenly Walt and Kim whispered, "What about Duke?" I felt guilty as I remembered that Duke was our dog when I was pregnant with Heather and when she was a small child.

Our sheepdog, Muffin, had been with us the longest and she was Heather's dog. Muffin had made such an impact on us that after her death from cancer, I wrote a book entitled *Muffin*. (Sometimes I feel that this book had a prophetic meaning for Heather.) I was so wrapped up in that focus that I had forgotten about our beautiful shepherd, Duke.

I remember wondering if dogs really could be on the other side (or heaven). But I was also surprised by the fact that George stated two (and only two) dogs. That was exactly correct. In our twenty-five years together, Walt and I have had only two dogs and never any cats before Heather got Jasmine. So, to us, this was a striking piece of information and something for me to consider.

On the ride home, the five of us spent the three hours discussing our reading. I was probably the most skeptical at that time due to my rigid fundamental approach to God and religion. Also, I was still angry with God as to what I was concluding to be a huge deception in my religious life.

As I mentioned before, it took me well over a year (with a lot more research) to truly appreciate the new picture that was forming. I would eventually come to see that there are different kinds of gifts given by the Spirit of God, yet they are all a part of the one.

Many people (ourselves included) have since tried to contact George, but have not been able to get through. My reasoning is that when the information is needed to come through, it will. Since George does not believe in calling up spirits, perhaps it is not a person's time to get a reading then. Or perhaps a person is supposed to be focusing on another avenue of development. Using prayer and meditation to seek guidance on this issue has helped many people.

I remember reading that Edgar Cayce had pointed out that each and every one of us has psychic ability to a certain degree. When asked how a person could become more psychic, Cayce admonished that the person should seek to become more spiritual. It is by becoming more spiritual that we come into closer contact with the One Spirit. Hence, the Spirit will give to each of us just what He determines will best suit our needs at that particular time.

Although it would take me quite a bit of time to appreciate this aspect of the Spirit, I am grateful for the blessing of that contact with Heather through George. It would eventually weave very well into the tapestry of my new beliefs.

8

Confrontation

"There is no fear in love. But perfect love drives out fear, because fear has to do with punishment. The one who fears is not made perfect in love."   *I John 4:18*

I H A D N O W reached a point where I knew that I had to come out of the "religious closet" and to stop living a double life. For almost twenty years, I had believed a lie and had existed in a prison of fear. I could not do this any more.

I had also been able to thoroughly research my own organization's background. To actually read the many false prophecies and to see the grip of fear that their people had been held under was very hard for me to swallow. Yet, in black and white, the proof was overwhelmingly there.

Although I hardly had all of the answers to this religious dilemma, I did know one thing for certain now. This organization was not the "only" true religious institution on the face of this earth as I had been brainwashed to believe. Of that, I was finally positive. I knew that I was no longer willing to stay in this organization and to dwell in fear.

Fortunately, my daughter, Kim, and a few close friends had also been willing to research the organization, and they, too, were prepared to leave. I sometimes wonder if I would have had the courage (or the desire) to leave if Kim had stayed in, and I had to give up my only other child. I am aware of people who know the facts about the organization, but still remain secretly inside because they know they will lose loved ones if they leave. I don't judge them; I pity them. But, most of all, I am grateful to God for revealing to me what He did and for the reassurance that death does not end a person's existence.

It was both amazing and unsettling for me to realize how little most of the people in the organization knew about its background and its false predictions. But what was even more amazing was the fact that no one wanted to know—including the elders. None of them wished to even read their own older literature to see the proof. I believe that it is the fear of being disfellowshiped by the organization and hence dying at Armageddon that prevents them from doing any independent research.

Fear is a very powerful emotion. Sad to say, it runs rampant in this world today. This creates undue attention on the body and the physical realm that we live in rather than focusing on the spiritual side of humanity. It is fear that produces many horrible and negative consequences on the earth. I believe that is why Jesus urged us to focus on the spirit when He said, "Do not be afraid of those who kill the body, but cannot kill the spirit." (Matthew 10:28) Why would He admonish us to consider this if the body and the spirit were the same thing?

By this time I had already read books on the importance of the mind/body connection. As I mentioned in chapter 6, there was a lot of material available. There were excellent research studies performed by the medical community on just how crucial our thought processes are to our illnesses and our cures. Many studies have indicated that people have totally cured themselves just by believing that they could cure themselves. There are also studies that suggest that illnesses can be caused by negative thinking. The field of psychiatry was born based on this concept.

Some people may consider the cures miraculous, while others view this as an ability programmed into the human brain. The fact is that there are many cases that prove that this phenomenon exists today.

In my case, my fear of death and my fear of a human-made concept of God and judgment had added tremendously to my grief and anxiety. I don't know why I have been finally freed from this fear, nor do I know why I have been blessed to experience the things I have. I just know that I am grateful to God for allowing me to gain this new freedom. I noticed the peace expanding in my life.

My readings and research have taught me a great truth. We are born alone and we die alone. Each birthing and dying experience is unique to the individual undergoing the experience. I was positive now that death was a transition to another dimension instead of an end-all experience.

I was also realizing that we are in a continuous relationship with God whether we are in a formal religion or not. Structure does not contain the essence of God. That is impossible. As soon as we define God, we limit God, because the concept is beyond human understanding.

This confrontation with my former religious organization, in spite of all the losses (and I do have losses), was also a very necessary part of my growth and healing. I remember hearing the expression, "Let go and let God." As I began to put this into practice over the years, I noticed that I moved more solidly into the stage of acceptance that grief counselors speak about. I remembered the Bible passage that said, "Whoever does not love does not know God, because God is Love." (I John 4:8)

Deep inside of me, I think I always knew that to be a fundamental truth. I believed that if we just strive sincerely to truly love our fellow humans, we couldn't possibly go wrong. My soul knew that to be true. I believe that is what Jesus was teaching us when He said, "For the entire Law stands fulfilled in one saying, namely: You must love your neighbor as yourself." (Galatians 5:14)

He did not say, "Join this group or join that group based on an intellectual understanding of God." He simply said, "Love your neighbor as yourself." I realize that this is not always easy to do. But I do believe it is the essential goal to strive for while we reside on the earth.

It wasn't easy to put this into practice when I went through my interrogations by the elders. It reached a point where my questioning and proofs were placing me in a position to be considered an "apostate" by them. I had the choice of either being disfellowshiped or resigning. I opted to resign so that people would know that it was my decision to leave and not that of the elders.

It is very empowering to take responsibility for one's own actions. I was very willing to do that. In spite of all the losses, I have never regretted that decision for a moment. Jesus had said, "You will come to know the truth and the truth will set you free." (John 8:32) Words can't explain the freedom and relief that I felt with this resignation.

This confrontation also enabled me to close one door and to watch a beautiful new door open for me. I believe it's important to speak of this confrontation, but not for me to dwell on the negative. I learned a lot from this experience.

A real positive factor here is that all of my readings and research have given me knowledge that is equivalent to a doctorate in philosophy or theology. The more I studied and learned, the more I could see how little humankind truly does know as fact. Therefore, this gives us tremendous potential for growth if we desire to seize the opportunity and not dwell on the negative.

As I see it, we are all born with a glass that is half full in our hands. How we choose to view the glass (either half full or half empty) will make us either psychologically healthy or unhealthy. But the choice is ours.

9

Did She Know?

"We speak of God's secret wisdom, a wisdom that has been hidden and that God destined for our glory before time began."   *I Corinthians 2:7*

I N   M Y   R E S E A R C H , I came across the concept of people knowing that they were dying. This is not an isolated concept and is found in both religious and medical literature. As I read about this, I began to remember and relive some important incidents in Heather's life.

One of these incidents occurred a few weeks before she died. It's important to mention that Heather was not expected to die. Far from it. She had been found to be cancer free and the only reason she was to finish her protocol (which involved three more treatments) was to insure her the best chance that the cancer would not return. So, technically, she was in remission at the time of the treatment that was given to her two weeks before she died.

We were on our way to the hospital for this five-day IV treatment and we were discussing her cat Jasmine. I get very attached to animals and had not wanted an animal after our sheepdog Muffin had died. But shortly after Heather was diagnosed, she wanted to get a pet, and I had a hard time refusing her because she was ill. So by the time this discussion took place, she had tried a Siamese cat (which she didn't seem to take to and gave away), a rabbit (again given away), and now her third animal, another cat.

Jasmine was really a beautiful cat and was working out very well. The problem was that she had become more of my responsibility than Heather's. That's exactly what had happened with Muffin. When Heather wasn't in the hospital, she would be off doing something with her friends. Therefore, it seemed that I had been assigned to take care of her cat. True, I did love the cat, but this was not the point.

As we were discussing this problem, I became annoyed that I now had the responsibility for another one of her animals that I hadn't really wanted in the first place. History seemed to be repeating itself. We had planned to do some traveling in the future, and I really didn't want the responsibility of caring for an animal at this time.

In the midst of this conversation, I asked her, "Why did you get the cat anyway?" She had been looking out the side window as I drove, and she just kept staring out that window. Then, she very quietly said to me, "So that you will have something to remember me by when I'm gone."

A terrible, odd feeling passed through me, and I felt myself gripping the steering wheel. I tried to make my voice sound casual as I said, "Why, do you plan on going somewhere?"

Her voice seemed vague and very tired. She just kept staring out the window, saying something like, "Well, you know that I may go on to college or get married or something;

and, besides, you know you love that cat."

I was very bothered by the discussion and quickly changed the subject. I did repeat this conversation to Walt, Kim, and some close friends. Everyone tried to reassure me that things would really be OK. Yet her words seemed to haunt me.

A few months after Heather died, several of us began to reflect on that conversation. We found it strange. But at the time of the conversation we had no idea what was really going on.

Another thing that I remembered was that a few days before her last treatment, she told me for the first time since her diagnosis that she did not want to have the next treatment. She even went so far as to ask me what I would do if she refused to go to have any more. I remembered crying and sitting on her bed, trying to make her understand how imperative it was for her to finish the full protocol assigned to her. Without it, she ran the risk of the cancer returning.

I remembered how she had been so sad that whole day and had kept crying. This was so out of character for her. She kept telling me that she was so sick of being sick and she wanted the treatments to end. I cried with her and my heart truly ached for her plight.

Her treatment protocol had run into some complications. She had her first operation on the primary site in September of 1989; this removed the rib that had the tumor. But in March of 1990, X-rays showed a suspicious site in the next rib over. This necessitated a second major surgery with more rib removal. Fortunately, this proved to be only scar tissue, but that second surgery was still a setback in her treatment plan.

Then, she had been accidentally chemically burned on her wrist from a leaking IV. This necessitated surgery with skin grafting to repair the wound and delayed her scheduled end of treatments. She was getting frustrated and tired.

To make matters worse, she had to have an emergency

appendectomy while she was hospitalized for wrist surgery. She had truly had her share of hospitals and treatments over the last year and a half.

Her treatments had been scheduled to end in July of 1990. But, here it was September and she faced three more intense IV treatments. I could understand her frustration and sadness.

Still, it was painful to see her so down. Heather had always been so upbeat during her illness and treatments that seeing her sadness truly brought sadness for us as well. This particular bout seemed to hang over all our heads during the next two weeks.

Then, all hell broke loose, as sadness turned to panic, to chaos, to horror, to death, and finally to insanity! Any parent who has lost a child will understand this insanity. Anyone who hasn't, God bless you; you are lucky that you don't understand.

I sometimes reflect on why she had to have that last round of chemotherapy. Why did the burn get out of control? Why was the infection that killed her not tended to immediately? But, more important, I wonder why she asked me if she could stop her treatments? She had never asked that before. Did she somehow subconsciously know what was soon to come? Did she know that her time here was about to be over?

There is a picture on Heather's bureau that she painted in art class about six months before she died. The painting was supposed to represent how she saw herself then and in the months to come. The picture reads from left to right and starts with a symbol of "no more tears."

This is followed by a heart floating in the sky which seems to be attached to something resembling an unraveling spool of thread. This is attached to a smiling sun with sunglasses on. It ends with a portrait of herself wearing a graduation cap and smiling. But instead of normal eyes, she had painted stars in her eyes where the pupils were to be. That is as far as she saw herself going at the time.

As I said, the picture was on her bureau for approximately six months before she died, and I had looked at it many times. It just seemed to be a nice representation of how she saw herself at that time. I hadn't given it any other thought then.

A few days after we buried Heather, I was in her room looking at that picture. An odd feeling rose up within me. I recalled a conversation that I had had with a nurse shortly after Heather died.

I had asked the doctors to remove the equipment from Heather as I couldn't stand to see her connected to all those machines. I just wanted to see her alone for a while. They complied with my wishes and took her off the machines and let me go in alone.

As I entered the room, a nurse was leaving and stopped to give her condolences. I was just staring toward Heather and I couldn't even say what the nurse looked like. I was noticing that Heather's lips were turned up in a smile and that her eyes were still half-opened and staring straight ahead. She had a look of "stars in her eyes." Her pupils actually looked like stars to me. I remember wondering how she could possibly have just come off a respirator and be smiling and looking so peaceful.

My horror turned into anger. I said to the nurse, "What do you people do? Push up the mouth into a smile to make the parents feel better?"

I remember how quietly she said, "No, we don't," and quickly left the room. I regret that now. But at the time, I really didn't believe her, and I was very angry.

My husband, my daughter Kim, and my cousin Pat also remarked at Heather's appearance. Every now and then, we all still mention how Heather looked to us that day, smiling with "stars in her eyes."

I had forgotten about that conversation until I stood there looking at the picture on her bureau. I thought, "Yes, my child, you made it through graduation and that was about it."

Her treatments had become so far delayed that she had not registered for the September semester of college. She had told me at that time that she didn't feel as if she belonged anyplace any more. All of her friends had now left for college, and September had truly begun with great sadness for all of us. We didn't know then that it would end in emotional devastation.

I remember trying to get her to enroll in a community college for a course or two so that she would be around people her age. I remember her telling me that she would only be wasting my money if she did that and that she did not want to go. I interpreted that to mean that she wasn't in the mood to apply herself. Perhaps she was really telling me so much more.

I remember, too, the morning that she died. My sister Fran, Kim, and I had been at the hospital all night. We would take turns sitting next to her and holding her hand to encourage her to go on. Walt was in such denial. He refused to believe that she could possibly die. He insisted that she would make it and went home prepared to go to work in the morning.

Although I was supposed to be trying to get some sleep since I had been up for two days straight, I felt compelled to go back in and sit by Heather's side. Fran and Kim tried to talk me into getting some sleep, but I just couldn't sleep.

At about 6:30 a.m., Fran and Kim went down to get some coffee and wanted me to go with them. I told them I would rather wait with Heather and asked them to bring me back some coffee when they returned. I just felt that I should stay.

There was a bathroom in this particular intensive care room and a nurse was stationed inside the room constantly attending to Heather. So if the nurse or I needed to use the bathroom, we would obviously use this one.

For some unknown reason, I stood up, looked at the

clock, and noticed that it was a few minutes before 7:00 a.m. I felt an urge to stretch my legs and to see if Fran and Kim were back yet. I walked out of that unit and into the hallway bathroom to wash my face. I had just entered the bathroom when I heard machines sounding and a commotion going on outside the door.

I came running out and tried to get back into the intensive care room. The medical personnel would not let me go in at that time. They told me that Heather had gone into cardiac arrest and that they were working on her. I hated myself for walking out of that room a few minutes before.

It wasn't until I got Heather's death certificate that I realized that the time of her death was actually 7:00 a.m. I have often agonized over the fact that I left for those few crucial minutes. What a horrible coincidence that she should die, alone, in those few minutes. One of us had constantly been by her side around the clock. Why did this have to happen during the few minutes that all three of us were out of the room? I got a possible answer two years later.

One day I came across a book called *Final Gifts*, written by two hospice nurses. This book explained that dying people often know the exact time of their deaths. Other death and dying books indicated this also. Some even said that people could control their time of death if loved ones needed to be there. If for some reason a loved one was not supposed to be present at the moment of death, the person dying would wait until that person left. I have often thought of this.

I had been with Heather the first time that she had died and I heard her dying words. I remembered the doctors actually telling me that she had died (on Monday afternoon of September 24). I even remember arguing with them and saying that this was impossible; it could not be true! I remember them gently trying to convince me that this was true.

Yet, in the midst of this dialogue, the intensive care nurse, Donna, came running over to me to tell me that she had brought Heather back and that Heather was now on a respirator. I remember asking her if it were possible for Heather to ever walk out of that hospital alive based on the condition she was now in.

Donna looked me directly in the eyes and said a firm, "Yes!" She then told me to compose myself if I wanted to be allowed back in with Heather. She warned me that she was on a respirator and asked if I could handle this.

The fact that she told me that it was possible for Heather to live and be all right was all that I needed to hear. I composed myself and went back in to be with Heather. This was when my heavy dialoguing and bargaining with God began.

I reflected back on that as I read *Final Gifts*. I wondered if God or Heather knew that I couldn't possibly bear to see her die a second time. I wonder, too, if Heather hadn't had a chance to see God on her "Road to Damascus" and been allowed to come back a second time to help me see the futility of her condition. At the end, had she chosen to stay with God?

Those hours spent watching her on that respirator and praying for her seemed like days and weeks to me. I aged tremendously during that ordeal. Was the time given as a teaching mechanism? I may not ever know in this dimension, but it certainly is a coincidence that she died during the few minutes that she was alone with her nurse.

Another odd thing happened on the day that she died. My mailbox contained a card from Heather's favorite cousin, Mike. Mike was in Florida, and Heather and her friend had planned to go to visit Mike as soon as her treatments were finished.

Mike knew she had been hospitalized when he sent her that card. That postcard was not, however, what Mike (a typical twenty-one-year-old guy) would send to Heather (his seventeen-year-old cousin). It was so obviously out of character for him.

The scene on the card was that of an empty chair in the midst of a beach where the sand and the water blended into the sky, which contained a few clouds. Although the card showed a very serene scene, no life at all could be felt in that card. Everyone, including his mother, Pat, remarked on the strangeness of that postcard. Mike himself said that he didn't know why he selected that card; he had actually wanted to send her a funny one, as he usually did. Did the universe know that she was dying?

I remember thinking how similar this scene was to the one that Heather had left for Walt and me just two weeks before she died. She had given us a card with a scene of the sky and some birds in flight. Nothing else was visible.

In the card, she told us that she knew how rough the past year and a half had been for all of us. She thanked us for having been by her side through the whole ordeal, and she told us how very much she loved us. I will treasure that card until the day I die. It is such a precious gift from her to us. Yet I still wonder, did she subconsciously know then what was about to happen?

I remembered the Friday night before she died as I held her on the way to the hospital. Her temperature on arrival was 104°. I remember thinking how hot she was as she lay against me. I remember how she kept going on and on about how much she loved us and appreciated all that we had done for her. But I also remember the fear as I noticed how hot she was. I knew I felt more fear for her at that time than I had ever felt before. I just didn't know why just then.

That conversation is another gift I will cherish from Heather until the day I die. Teenage years can be rough. Hers were no exception. For parents to hear words of endearment from their teenager is a gift beyond compare. I thank Heather with all my heart and again wonder, did she know?

On the day of her funeral something happened that brought laughter to some through their tears. We had come back to our house with some friends after the funeral. Every time that someone would use the ice machine, it would give out crushed ice. It didn't matter if the setting was on cubes or crushed. It would only produce crushed ice.

Heather and I had this thing about the ice machine. She loved crushed ice. I hated all those little chips in my water. I usually wasn't paying attention at the ice machine, and as I filled my glass, I'd realize that I was getting crushed ice. I would become annoyed and dump it out and put the setting on cubes. I would then holler out, "Heather, you did it again!" She would laugh.

She would do the same thing. When she came to get ice, she would be talking before she would realize that her glass was half full of ice cubes. Then she would dump her glass out and look at me annoyed. I'd then laugh.

So the day of her funeral, when everyone got crushed ice regardless of the setting, people began to remark, "Heather must be here." Of course, I didn't believe any of that sort of thing at the time, but if it made people laugh through their tears, I figured it was OK to say it.

This phenomenon of crushed ice lasted for a few weeks and then fixed itself. We had a repair man look at it, but he couldn't find anything wrong. He had no idea why the ice maker was acting in this manner. We just sort of accepted the experience, as it was the least of our worries then.

Yet, to this day, people will remember that incident and remark that Heather must have been there that day. With the understanding that I have now, I believe that she was.

10

The Sequins

"I am so sure of you . . . I am still full of courage, I am running over with joy."   *II Corinthians 7:4*

TEN MONTHS OR so after the calla-lily incident, another strange thing happened in our home. I was making coffee in our upstairs sitting room (directly over Heather's room). Walt was still sleeping. The sun's rays were coming in through the sliding-glass door and an object was shining on the floor. It looked like a piece of blue metallic paper and I walked over to pick it up. I was absolutely stunned!

It was a thread with two blue sequins on it and it was from Heather's prom gown. I knew that Heather's prom gown was sealed in a bag in her closet downstairs in her bedroom. It had been there since the day after her prom, almost two years now.

I knew that there were a few sequins at the bottom of a prom souvenir glass in her bedroom on her bureau. I wondered how the sequins could have gotten upstairs and onto this rug. I had vacuumed the rugs just the day before and no one had been in the house over the last few days.

I ran downstairs to see the souvenir glass and thought that perhaps the cat had knocked it over. But how could the cat get the sequins upstairs?

The glass sat in the same position and nothing else on that cluttered bureau was disturbed. It was highly unlikely that one (we now had two) of the cats would be graceful enough to jump up onto the bureau, put its paw in the glass, reach down to the bottom of the glass, extract two sequins, and, without moving anything, be able to jump back down and bring the sequins across the entire bottom floor, up a flight of fourteen stairs, around a corner, and into the sitting room.

How would the cat carry the sequins? Would it be by paw or by mouth? Although I was trying to look for a logical answer, I knew deep inside of me that this was not the answer. I wondered what the meaning of it was.

I remembered that Heather had never been upstairs with her gown on. All of the rugs had been cleaned twice professionally since her death. I also had vacuumed all the rugs hundreds of times since her death. So, I wondered what the explanation and meaning could be.

I discussed this with Walt and some of our friends. We all agreed that there was no logical explanation. We also did not know what the significance of this might be.

That incident took place on a Wednesday morning. On Friday morning, I was putting my running shoes on while sitting on the edge of my bed. I looked down and saw a single blue sequin right next to the bottom of our bed along the side that I sleep on. I gasped!

It was approximately 11:00 a.m. and I was alone in the house. I could not even imagine how another sequin could have gotten out of that glass and all the way upstairs. This time, it was even farther than the one on Wednesday morning. I remembered that I had vacuumed both Wednesday and Thursday with much more attention than I normally would have when I vacuum. Since I remembered the Wednesday sequin appearance, I guess I was looking for other clues.

I picked up the sequin and ran downstairs into Heather's room. I looked at the bureau. It was exactly the same. It just had more dust. Nothing was disturbed. No marks were in the dust. What was this all about?

I felt a surge of excitement go through my body. I called a few close friends to tell them of this second sequin. One of them, Marilyn, told me to count the sequins in the glass and to write the number down on a piece of paper. I said, "Good idea!"

Of course, no one had an explanation. Everyone knew that my cats can get wild and crazy and, therefore, didn't believe that they could be graceful enough to accomplish such a feat. We wondered more about the meaning of this than we did about the how of the matter.

I counted the sequins, which totaled six in all, and wrote this on a piece of paper. I was very excited. I went out for an hour-long walk; all the time, I kept thinking about the sequins appearing. Heather was heavy on my mind.

I came back in and tried to get busy. I had friends coming in for dinner that night. Two of these friends, Jim and Judy, were working on Heather's scholarship with me and I couldn't wait to see them to tell them what had happened. Maybe they could provide some further insight.

It was getting close to dinner time, and I still had not vacuumed the downstairs Oriental rugs (which were purchased approximately a year after Heather died). I was on the last runner near the front door when my eye caught the shining object. Another blue sequin was lying on the Oriental runner. I began to laugh and cry at the same time.

I looked up over my head almost expecting to see

Heather laughing. I called out, "Heather, what are you try-ing to tell me?"

In my mind's eye, I could picture that silly grin on her face. She always had a great sense of humor and loved to play tricks on me. Laughing and crying at the same time was an odd experience for me.

I had remembered telling Gene that I knew I would never be able to laugh again. I almost felt that if I did laugh, it would be disrespectful to her memory. How can you ever laugh again after your child dies? Impossible. Yet, here I was, laughing and crying at the same time. Still, I was filled with such wonder.

I took Marilyn's advice and put a number seven on my piece of paper. I walked (not ran this time) into Heather's room just to look at the glass on her bureau. The bureau was still exactly the same as it had been for months.

I no longer doubted or questioned that this was beyond the dimension of human possibility. I seemed more focused on what it meant than I was on how it had happened.

I stood in her room. I quietly whispered, "I love you, baby; are you here?" No one answered. I felt overwhelmed with such love for her, and although the tears were still running down my face, the sadness was now somehow different. I felt different. I'm not sure how; I just know I felt changed, perhaps even peaceful.

I put that seventh sequin into the souvenir glass and be-gan finishing dinner. My guests arrived within the hour. Again, no one could explain what had happened, and no one thought my cats were that talented. I had crossed out the original six and the paper now had a number seven. That seven is still there today. Whatever moved those se-quins has never moved them again. And, to this day, I can't tell you what the meaning of it really is.

Coincidentally, though, something did arrive that night that became new food for thought and perhaps another dot on my spiritual canvas.

I had ordered the book *A Window to Heaven* by Dr. Diane Komp, a pediatric oncologist at Yale. I had read about this book in the Candlelighters Newsletter and my friend, Ginny, had ordered it for me from the bookstore where she had been working. Since it had just arrived that day, Ginny brought the book with her when she came to dinner that night. I didn't have a chance to look at it until Saturday morning.

As I perused the book, I came to page 19 which had an excerpt from *The House in Paris* by Elizabeth Bowen. It read in part, "With three or more . . . to be three is to be in public, you feel safe."

This seemed to really stand out in my mind because I wondered what the significance of the three sequins was supposed to mean. I kept thinking, "Why not one or two or even more? Why just three?" And why over a period of three days? Was this some kind of a cryptic code? I still don't have an answer for this, but I'm sure that was why the passage seemed to stand out in my mind at that time.

Later that day, Cynthia and Elwood stopped by to visit. We talked about the three sequins, and I showed Cynthia the book with the excerpt from page 19 about the significance of three. She had never heard of the book and took it from me and scanned it. She asked me if she could borrow it after I had finished reading it. Of course, I told her that she could.

We talked about the sequins and we agreed that there probably was no answer in this dimension. Elwood told me that I should stop trying to figure everything out and to just accept it as a miracle without an explanation. This was a very interesting remark coming from the newly retired major of the state police. I had to smile as I said to him, "You're right, I have to stop trying to have an answer for everything."

I finished the book the next morning, Sunday. It left me feeling very peaceful and full of hope. I went out to do my daily walk. I wanted to think and to meditate.

It was a beautiful sunny day. As I walked, I reflected on the events of the past few days and the material I had been reading. I began to realize that I wasn't thinking so much at that point as I was more interested in how I seemed to be feeling.

I began to notice an overpowering sense of euphoria building inside of me. I was truly overwhelmed with such pure joy that I felt as if my feet were hardly touching the pavement. Joy seemed to permeate my whole body.

Joy was an emotion I probably had not experienced in almost twenty years. It was never really a word that was found in my vocabulary. Yet, I was filled with such extreme joy that I thought I would burst. Tears were running down my face, and I was glad that I had my sunglasses on.

I kept telling myself that I had experienced a miracle, and here I was still trying to analyze it. I had to laugh as I remembered Elwood telling me yesterday this very same thing.

I scolded myself for still being so skeptical. I knew Elwood was right and that I should just accept it. I told myself to accept it with thanks to God for this miracle. This thought process was rapidly taken over by the most incredible joy that I have ever experienced in my life. I just let go and bathed in the feeling.

I finally walked back home feeling so elated that it seemed as if I had just stepped off a cloud. As I entered my house, I noticed that my answering machine light was on. It was Cynthia. I called her back.

She said to me, "You won't believe what just happened at my church." I really couldn't imagine what had happened.

She told me that her church had a visiting pastor that day who had come up to the podium and held up the book *A Window to Heaven*. He then explained to the congregation that his discourse was to be on "Miracles."

Cynthia said that she just sat there awestruck, thinking, "My God, that's the same book that Geri just read from yesterday, and we had even discussed miracles. What a coincidence this is! I'll have to call her as soon as I get home and tell her."

Little did she know that as she was sitting in church thinking her thoughts, I was walking on the road thinking my thoughts—and we were thinking about the same thing. Talk about synchronicity! I certainly had no way of controlling the sequins, the arrival of the book, or the visiting pastor's discourse. There are millions of books in this world. Why that book and on that day?

The reading of that book affected me for several reasons. Timing was certainly one of them. But the fact that Dr. Komp is a highly respected pediatric oncologist from Yale is another. This was the medical profession acknowledging that there is another dimension that science has yet to explain. Even the hard-core skeptics have to take note of that.

Also, coincidentally, I had just finished reading *Love, Medicine, and Miracles* by Dr. Bernie Siegel. He, too, is a highly respected oncologist from Yale. So, to come across Dr. Komp's book in the manner in which I did and with this timing was certainly making the unbelievable now more believable.

As I mentioned earlier, there were a lot of books written about the mind/body connection from the medical/psychological community, as well as from the spiritual/religious fields, that were helping me to realize how much was really going on in the world.

The manner in which I was introduced to these books was sometimes as important as the book itself. "When the student is ready, the teacher arrives" was really being applied in my life. I began to take notice of how I got my books, when I got my books, and from whom I got my books. This proved to be very helpful and interesting. Things that I once viewed as only coincidental I now considered to be divine timing. The concept of synchronicity had really become obvious in my life.

I became aware that I was connected to something greater than I could comprehend. I felt I was being drawn or moved along by something that I could not explain. As I considered this aspect in my life, I couldn't help but think about the significance that a rose has in my life.

11

The Rose

"... God has accepted your prayers ... and he has remembered you."   Acts 10:4

A S S O O N A S someone mentions the word *rose* my mind goes into gear. For me, the rose means several things. It began with the words to the song "The Rose."

Heather was not particularly fond of that song. I loved it. Every time it played on the radio, I would turn up the radio full blast. In those days, I tended to focus on the parts of the song that depict a sense of loneliness and futility about life, and for some reason this would evoke a feeling of sadness in me and sometimes even tears. I found the song to be very moving.

Heather would poke fun at me and tease me saying, "Oh,

Ma, it's just a song." Although I had never seen the movie, that song really affected me.

One day, a few months after Heather died (and before I did a lot of heavy research), my cousin Celia invited me to lunch at her house. Although I was very reclusive at that time, I accepted the invitation and drove to her house.

As I pulled into her driveway, "The Rose" began playing on the car radio. I burst into tears and began to think of Heather immediately. I waited until the song finished, dried my eyes, and went in to visit. I was very uncomfortable with my grief at this point, and I did not mention the incident to Celia.

We had a nice lunch and sat and talked for a while. She knew that I was very sad. I remember telling Celia how hard it was to have faith in the unseen and how I would love to be able to just open the sky for a moment to see if Heather was there and all right.

Celia sat quietly thinking about what I had just said. She then got up and went to her bookcase. She came back with a card about St. Theresa of the Roses. She explained to me that some people claimed that when they said this prayer on the card, they would receive an answer in the form of a rose. She said that the rose could be real or that it could be a picture or a card or something like that, but that they would receive a form of the rose. The receiving of this flower would be an indication that God had answered their prayer.

She proceeded to explain to me that she personally had never experienced this, but that she knew of people who had received an answer to their prayers in this manner. She asked me what I wanted to know from God.

I told her that I wondered if Heather existed as a spirit and if she was really OK. She told me to phrase this question into the prayer and to wait for an answer.

This entire conversation was odd to begin with when one considers that she was a Roman Catholic who knew that my religious organization did not believe in this. Just having this conversation with her and saying the prayer could get me disfellowshiped as an "apostate." Although my mind seemed to be aware of this fact, my heart did not seem to care about that.

Desperate for some kind of answer, I thought that I would give this prayer a try but that I would keep it quiet. I asked Celia not to tell anyone that she had given me this card. Though she didn't quite understand, she agreed to keep it confidential.

I said the prayer in the car before I left her driveway and continued praying about this all the way home. I cried to God; I begged Him for an answer. I begged Him to hear my prayer even if I weren't Catholic, and I begged Him to give me a sign that Heather was OK. I had quite a tearful conversation with Him on that fifteen-minute ride home.

I was in my house for about five minutes when the song "The Rose" came on the radio. I stopped short. My mind seemed to be in slow gear as the thought went through my head, "O my God, You didn't just give me a rose; You gave me 'The Rose.'"

I began to sob as the words of the song played loudly in the house. I kept saying, "My God, my God, are You really answering my prayer?" I really couldn't believe this to be true.

I called my cousin Celia and asked her if the answer could come in the form of a song. She said that she really didn't know, but that she didn't see why not. Although I don't know of anyone else whose answer came in this way, I do believe today that this was an answer.

In those days, I was still too afraid to believe that it was more than a coincidence. Now when I review this incident, I realize that coincidence could not have been the explanation. If so, it would have to be a very startling one, indeed, for several reasons.

First, I had not mentioned to Celia that "The Rose" had been playing on the radio when I pulled into her driveway. She also did not know how I felt about that song.

Second, only Walt, Heather, and I (and God) knew about my deep attachment to that song at this time in my life. Further, it was Heather who always teased me about it.

Third, I had never heard of St. Theresa of the Roses nor had I heard of the prayer and the phenomenon attached to it. Further, being a Jehovah's Witness would certainly have prevented me from even considering this experiment with that prayer, nor would I normally have had the desire to do that.

Fourth, I had the same radio station on in my car as I always do in my home. "The Rose" is an old song, and I don't often hear it. For me to hear that same song within a few hours on the same radio station is rare indeed—especially since this station prides itself on not repeating songs.

Fifth, to actually say the prayer and then to hear the song (no matter what station was involved) would be pretty incredible in itself. Only fifteen minutes had elapsed from the prayer to the song. That, in itself, is pretty amazing.

Coincidence? I choose to believe otherwise. Since the word *synchronicity* was not in my vocabulary at that time, I viewed this as a unique set of coincidences, as well as an answer to my prayer.

Celia and I have told this story to many people over the last few years. They all find it pretty incredible, too. I am not the only one to claim that a prayer to St. Theresa of the Roses was answered in some way by a rose. Sadly enough, I would request this prayer once again in the future regarding Walt's brother, and I would also have it answered.

I grew to appreciate and understand this incident more and more as the months went by. Since I was so narrow in my thinking at that time, I had no basis for understanding what really may have been happening. I was too consumed with my grief and too fearful of my religious structure then to consciously pursue this phenomenon. True, I did find it rather amazing when it happened, but it would take time for the understanding to penetrate.

This phenomenon with the rose did not end there. One day as I was listening to a tape by Dr. Weiss on *Many Lives, Many Masters,* I heard him mention the name of Dr. Bernie Siegel. As soon as I heard it, I remember saying to my husband, "Why is that name familiar?"

He didn't seem to know. Suddenly, I remembered that Heather had a copy of a book by Dr. Siegel, and it was the very book that Dr. Weiss was referring to in his tape.

I turned off the tape recorder and went into Heather's room to look for the book. I found not one but two copies of the book *Love, Medicine, and Miracles.* But it was the cover of the book that really got to me. It had a rose on it! (So do his next two books and his tape set.) I have no idea what the rose signifies to Dr. Siegel, but it must be meaningful to him.

I felt sad as I held the copies of that book. I knew that Heather must have touched these books. I wondered if she had ever read them. I wondered who gave them to her. I felt odd and sad at the same time. I remember saying to Walt, "I think that I'm supposed to read this book."

I felt suddenly overwhelmed with feelings and thoughts of Heather. I stopped what I was doing and decided to go upstairs and scan through the book. I wasn't even sure what I was looking for; I just knew that I needed to read this book.

As I became enthralled with the book, Walt was digging things out of the basement. He brought up a large portfolio of Heather's work that she had put away the summer before she died. He opened it and began going through her works. Suddenly, he began to cry. He told me to come and see something.

I went downstairs to see an 18" x 20" charcoal sketch that Heather had made of a rose. I burst into tears as I exclaimed how beautiful a rose Heather had given to us.

I remembered her sketching it one day before the end of her senior year. I could visualize her with no hair and sitting in her night shirt sketching a rose that someone had sent to her. At that time, she didn't think it turned out very good.

But I kept telling her how perfect and beautiful it really was. This sketch was later matted and framed and hangs on our dining room wall to this day. Everyone remarks on how beautiful it really is.

As I stood there looking at the drawing, I wondered how I could have forgotten about this. I touched the paper carefully as if I were touching a part of her soul. Although happy to have retrieved this precious piece of her art, Walt and I both cried over what could have been and what we believed in our hearts should have been. The whys still remain with me to this day.

The rose has truly taken on a special meaning for me. Even the song has become a teaching mechanism for me. As I said before, I used to focus on the sad part of the song and cry. Now, I seem to see the spiritual meaning to this song and feel uplifted.

This song also enabled me to see a side of myself that I had not been conscious of before. Some of the words focus on the impact that fear can have in a person's life. My attention seemed to be drawn to the fact that the fear of dying could, in a sense, prevent one from truly experiencing the gift of living. In a way, this could almost negate one's life. It was these words that now became dominant in my mind.

Had I missed the point of the song? Worse yet, had I lived in such fear that I had really missed the point of life? It was almost as if I had never heard this part of the song before. Yet, as I look back now, I had been so narrowly focused and dwelled in such fear that, in essence, I had been too afraid to really live.

Heather, on the other hand, had loved life. She had wanted to participate in the experience of life on this earth. So, she lived her life and truly was a wonderful participant in this gift of life.

I had been far too fearful a person. I had feared God. I had feared death. Hence, I had missed the point of life. Was God now trying to tell me something?

I also thought of the words in the song that picture the seasons of the year. When we look out on a winter day, it is sometimes hard to believe that spring will come and life will be evident again. We wonder how any seeds could actually survive through the bitter cold.

That concept in the song has become highly symbolic to me now. I think the winter symbolizes death; the spring refers to the resurrection; and the sun's love refers to God's love. The seed that becomes the rose, to me, means the spirit.

This may not mean the same thing to other people (and that's OK), but to me this song became quite a teaching mechanism with Heather being the catalyst. I am now focused in a different way. The rose is a symbol of that new focus and understanding.

Time would again reveal to me that the rose wasn't yet finished with its enlightenment process. To this day, the rose interacts symbolically in my life and at such appropriate times.

12

Songs

"... as you teach and admonish one another with all wis-
dom, and as you sing psalms, hymns and songs with grati-
tude to God."   *Colossians 3:16*

TWO SONGS, IN addition to "The Rose," are very
significant in our life with Heather. A few months before
Heather died, "Don't Know Much" by Linda Ronstadt and
"When I'm Back on My Feet Again" by Michael Bolton were
very popular. Both of these songs remind me of Heather. They
seemed to play frequently during the time of Heather's wake
and funeral days, and we dedicated both of them to her.

Sometimes we may like a song and sing it a lot; yet, we
may never really hear all of the words. That's how it was for
me with "When I'm Back on My Feet Again." I would always
say to Heather, "That's your song to the world."

I, of course, was focused on the fact that she would get back on her feet again after her treatments. As I think back on this, she never did say too much when I said that to her.

One day in August of 1990, Walt and I were on our boat with his cousin, Shelia, and her children. This song began to play on the radio. Normally, I would say, "That's Heather's song to the world."

I remember suddenly being consumed with this over-whelming feeling of sadness. I broke into uncontrollable sobs which really took Shelia and Walt by surprise. Shelia tried to console me, yet I remember feeling as if something bad were going to happen. I didn't know why I felt that way; I just suddenly felt like that when the song began playing.

We even talked about the fact that Heather's last scan had shown her to be cancer free and that the remaining treatments were just a precautionary measure. In my mind, I knew this and really believed it. Yet I still had this over-whelming sense of dread come upon me for some unknown reason.

Heather died approximately one month after that incident and very unexpectedly. It wasn't until sometime after her funeral that I became focused on the other words in this song.

A friend of ours, Mary, referred to that song and asked me if I had ever really listened closely to all the words. I thought that I had, but the next time that this song played, I knew what she was talking about.

The words referencing the children laughing and the sweet light of heaven suddenly became very obvious. A funny feeling came over me. I wondered if Heather had noticed those words and that was why she never answered me when I connected the song to her. Did we both know deep down, perhaps on a subconscious level, that Heather would only be back on her feet again when she accessed the light of heaven?

The other song, "Don't Know Much," would just tear my

heart out. I remember driving Heather home from the hospital one day when this song came on the radio. She was still feeling ill from the treatments and was not having a very good day. She looked so white and pale as she lay back against the seat of the car.

When the song came on the radio, I felt overwhelmed with feelings of such love and compassion for her that tears ran down my face. I reached over and grabbed her knee and gently shook it. I said, "I love you, Heather, and I am so sorry that you are sick."

She looked at me with her stark white face and those beautiful blue eyes and gave me the sweetest half-smile. She quietly said, "I know, Mom; it's OK."

But my heart was breaking inside for my child. It's sheer hell to watch your child suffer and not be able to do a damned thing about it. My focus during the song was on my love for her. That song still means that to me, but has expanded to mean much more.

As the years passed and we arrived at her third memorial anniversary, the expanded meaning was really making itself known. We decided to use a phrase from that song for her memorial remembrance in the newspaper, and it was this new and expanded meaning that was significant when we chose this.

I can't count the times that I have screamed, cried, and begged the universe to give me answers to the why of her death and to where she was. But the more I was reading and learning, the fewer concrete answers I actually had.

The song indicated to me what I was coming to realize about myself. I really didn't know much about the workings of this universe. Yet the one thing I did know was how very much I loved her. This song really does state a fundamental truth about life.

Love was all I needed to know. Too simple? Perhaps not. The Bible says, "Whoever does not love does not know God, because God is Love." (I John 4:8)

I must have read and quoted that scripture close to a thousand times over a twenty-year period. But that concept had never seemed enough. It was too simple. I needed an intellectual concept of God.

So I accumulated tons of facts (no faith, just facts).

I carried these facts around me like a suit of armor. I had all the answers to life and death until Heather died. Then, this "book faith" that I had acquired suddenly didn't mean a damned thing. It wasn't even real. I had facts all right, but I learned that I never really had any faith.

Jesus' main focus was love. When asked what the greatest of the commandments was, Jesus answered, "One must love God and love his neighbor as himself." (Matthew 22:36-40) In this way, one could fulfill the law and the prophecies. Again, a simple answer, but it is not always easy to put this into practice.

I do know that these songs cause me to focus instantly on Heather and my love for her. I have come to believe that there is a lot we will never know in this lifetime; knowledge is not the answer here. Love is what survives—even death. It is in the act of loving that we become Christlike. Love is not a feeling; it's an action taken by us, whether it be in thought or in deed. We sometimes forget that thinking is an activity that can motivate us to do (or not to do) something. Thinking about love is not only important; I believe it is essential.

13

The Memphis Experience

Jesus looked at them and said, "With man this is impossible, but with God all things are possible." Matthew 19:26

IN JANUARY OF 1993, I had an interesting dream. In the dream, I was talking to Elvis Presley. I acknowledged that I knew that he was dead. I also told him that it was very difficult to sometimes understand information about the other side and how different people seem to have different ideas about life after death.

He gave me a very interesting answer. He told me that the people on the earth were limited and imperfect. He explained that even though we may be given one hundred percent perfectly correct information from the other side, the problem would be in the receiving (not transmitting) end.

He further explained that since the receivers were imperfect (or limited), the information would not be able to be collated and disseminated in a one hundred percent accurate way on the earth. He told me that this was not due so much to dishonest attempts to deceive, but it was more in the inability of the receiver to perfectly take in and interpret information. I pictured a radio station that wasn't coming in clearly and had static making it difficult to understand.

I told this to my friend Carol, who now lives in Mississippi, and we both laughed. We thought it was very interesting information, but mostly we found it amusing at the time.

We wondered why Elvis was the symbol. I didn't recall having seen or heard anything about him in quite some time, and she couldn't think of anything that would make the timing significant. So we weren't sure what he could represent in that dream.

Since Carol had been after me to come down and visit her, she teased me and said that maybe I was being directed to visit her and that we could go up and visit Graceland. We both got a good laugh out of that line of logic. I told her that I would give the idea some serious thought and perhaps I could visit her in the summer.

A few months later, I called to book my flight. I wanted to go from Monday through Friday (June 7-11) because Walt was busy with his work during the week and free on the weekends. I hated to leave him alone.

When I called to make a reservation, the agent told me that it would be almost triple the fare if I didn't take a Saturday overnight. I, therefore, decided to go from Wednesday through Sunday, June 9-13. My main thought in booking these dates was to save money.

June 9 finally arrived. I got up early and went downstairs into Heather's room to say a goodbye. Since visiting her room was a daily habit, I knew I would miss not having her familiar objects around me. It was a big step for me to fly alone and leave Walt home. I had never done this before and I felt anxious about it.

As soon as I entered her room, I noticed that an 8-1/2" x 11" picture of her (in a gold frame) had been turned completely sideways. Instead of facing the door, it was now facing the wall with the 45" x 45" contemporary design Heather had made (the same wall that Walt had seen her pass into over two years before).

The picture was on top of a newspaper article about her, on a very small, cluttered night stand. I looked to see if the paper was rumpled or moved. Nothing else seemed to have been touched. To get the picture in this position, it would have to be picked up and turned. Yet no one had been in the house over the last few days and I had been in her room just yesterday. Although I felt that this was of the paranormal, I went upstairs to ask Walt if he had moved it the previous night.

He told me that he had not moved the picture. In fact, he had not been in her room for several days. We both thought that she must be trying to tell us something, but we did not know what.

Suddenly, the date of June 9 entered my mind. Why did this seem so important? I remembered that we had flown to Hawaii with Heather on "A Wish Come True" trip a few days after her graduation in June, but I wasn't sure of the exact date.

I took out the Hawaii album and I looked at the ticket date. Sure enough, June 9, 1990, was on the ticket. Tears welled up in my eyes. I remembered that I had been so focused on Heather's illness at the time that I didn't even enjoy the Hawaiian trip; no wonder I hadn't remembered the date.

Yet Heather had loved the trip and it had been such a boost to her spirits. She had talked about the trip until the day that she died (some three-and-a-half months later).

I suddenly felt guilty for being alive, and I felt so sad that

Heather wasn't with me. I thought to myself that only twice in my life had I flown on June 9. The first time was with Heather and Walt, and now this time I would fly alone.

I still couldn't get the significance of the picture being turned sideways, facing a different direction. I smiled a bit as I noticed that I was still trying to analyze things to get an exact answer. Yet there really wasn't one.

I arrived in Mississippi and met Carol as scheduled. As soon as we started walking toward her car, I began to tell her about the picture and the June 9 date. She stopped and looked at me quietly. She said that she, too, had encountered an unusual thing that morning.

She told me that she had a rose bush that had never bloomed since she began living in Mississippi. She said that she had walked by it several times over the last few days and had laughingly said to it, "Why don't you bloom for Geri."

She knew how special a rose was to me. Her husband, John, and her son, Jason, had laughed at her when she told them what she had said to the bush. Jason said, "Ma, I think you've lost it." She laughed, too.

Yet the day that I was to arrive, she walked outside and noticed that one rose had bloomed. She couldn't believe it! Neither could John nor Jason. They called it just a coincidence. Carol couldn't wait to show me this rose.

When we arrived at her house, we looked at the rose. It was a beautiful pink with traces of white in it. I told her that Heather had a silk rose on her bed that was the same color as this one. Someone had given it to her for graduation, and it now rested across the two pillows on her bed. This was truly a remarkable coincidence!

Carol had no idea what color the rose was supposed to be since the bush had never bloomed while she lived there. Also, she had not been aware at all of Heather's graduation gifts (some three years ago). So for the two roses to be almost the same color was quite uncanny.

We walked around outside for a while, and I admired the

beautiful landscape, flowers, and trees in their yard. We then went into the house and she began to show me around. It was really lovely, since Carol has a knack for decorating.

When we entered Jason's room, I stopped short. Facing me was the identical picture and frame that had been moved in Heather's room that morning. The whole 8-1/2" x 11" picture and frame were identical. It was as if it had been transported across the miles and was here with me now. I gasped.

I asked Carol where Jason had gotten the picture and the frame. She explained that on Heather's funeral day, Jason had wanted a copy of that picture of Heather, and so I had let Carol take it to make him a copy.

Since that was almost three years ago, I had forgotten about it. So many people had borrowed pictures and negatives from us to make copies that I really didn't remember who had which picture of Heather in their homes. Even more enlightening was the origin of the frame.

Carol explained to me that she was the one who had bought both frames. She said that because I had been so upset and didn't want to go shopping, she had bought me the frame as a gift. At that time, she bought Jason the same frame. I was not previously aware of that fact.

I had forgotten that it was Carol who had bought me the frame. She had also purchased the frame for the 5" x 7" picture that had been turned over on the night of the "Calla-lily incident."

To stand at Jason's door and to see the identical picture and frame was quite startling. Was there a message here? The same thing, but in a different location. Could it be that Heather was the same person, but in a different location (heaven)? Again my mind was racing for answers.

This journey had started out strangely enough, but we would eventually find out that it wasn't over yet. This visit would begin to show me how connected we all are to one another.

It was wonderful to see Carol, John, and Jason. Jason and Heather had been such good friends, and I knew that he really missed her. I was glad to be with them all and I felt very peaceful there. Maybe Heather was here, after all.

The Saturday before I left, Jason wanted to take us to Memphis to visit Graceland. I remembered the dream of Elvis, and Carol and I began to laugh. Jason just listened to us and shook his head and smiled.

As we toured the mansion, I pointed to all the books that Elvis had been reading. Jason listened as I pointed to a book and told Carol that Elvis, too, seemed to be a seeker.

I felt sad as I left Carol at the airport. I told her I would call when I got home, and I boarded the plane. We had a layover in Chicago. This was a sad stop for me. I remembered that when we flew to Hawaii, we had also had a layover in Chicago. I closed my eyes for a moment, and I could picture Heather in the airport with me some three years before.

I remembered how we had all joked then about my father.

He had always been amused by my mother's method of giving people directions and would remark, "Oh sure, they'll get there all right, but by way of Chicago." As Walt, Heather, and I mentioned it that day, I remember saying, "Well, Daddy, we are finally in Chicago."

This was the second time in my life that I had sat in the Chicago airport. I sadly whispered, "Hey, Daddy, I'm in Chicago again, but where in the universe are you guys? Is Heather with you?" I could feel the tears well up in my eyes. I felt so nostalgic. I would be glad to get home and see Walt again. I missed him greatly.

I called Carol when I got home. She told me that when she had returned from the airport, she noticed that the rose had fallen from the bush. Another coincidence.

A few days later, my nieces stopped over to visit. I began excitedly to tell them of my experiences. When I mentioned June 9, Lori looked at me seriously and said, "Aunt Geri, wasn't that Heather's first surgery date? Wasn't that the date of the biopsy on her rib?"

A cold feeling went through me as my mind raced back in time. I had repressed so much of Heather's illness and death that it actually shocked me that I could possibly have forgotten this piece of the horror story. But I had.

I told Lori that I would check my journal to be sure, but I already knew that she was correct. How our minds struggle to survive! It's really a necessity to refocus eventually or one would end up in an institution. I also believe that God was trying to tell me to focus in another direction; otherwise, I would have immediately remembered the June 9 surgery. Instead, I thought of the Hawaiian trip—a trip that brought Heather tremendous happiness.

As my nieces and I continued this conversation, they wanted me to show them which picture had been turned. Five of us entered her room.

We were halfway across the room when suddenly the rose on Heather's bed rolled slowly down from the pillows and onto the bed. Kathy and her son, Kevin, were looking directly at the bed, while Lori (holding Ethan) and I were looking more toward the corner of the room at Heather's picture. Lori and I could see something moving just as we heard both Kathy and Kevin gasp. Ethan jumped in Lori's arms and made a "squealing" sound.

As I looked at Kathy and Kevin, I noticed that their eyes seemed as big as saucers. They pointed at the bed, and Lori and I realized that the rose was the object we saw moving. Kevin said, "Aunt Geri, did you see that?"

Kathy could hardly speak and sort of stammered out, "It just rolled gently down from the pillows and then stopped. That's really weird!"

The way the rose had been positioned across the two pillows would have made it impossible for it to roll down on its own. There were no windows open, and no one was even close to this heavy-framed king-sized bed. That rose had been positioned there for almost three years now, and the stem had even become bowed in (not flat) from all this time. Something had to move that rose. Yet, we all saw it move on its own accord before our very eyes. We still wonder what made Ethan "squeal." (He was eleven months old then.)

Walt heard our excited voices and came into the room. We explained to him what had happened. He agreed that there was just no way that the rose could have moved by itself; yet, it had.

As I mentioned before, the rose was the same color as Carol's mystery rose in Mississippi. What could this mean? Was there some connection? Perhaps the same picture in two locations and the same-color rose in two locations were telling me that Heather was really present but just in another location.

Or perhaps she was just letting us know that she was still around checking in with us. Maybe she had just wanted to greet her cousins whom she so dearly loved. I can't be sure, but this wasn't the end of it.

Shortly after I had experienced the dream of Elvis Presley, I had been introduced to a physician (through Gene) who had recently lost her daughter. Celina and I became instant friends. We both felt as if we knew each other from before. We had a lot in common. The saddest connection was that each of us had lost our daughters. As a result, we both were seeking answers.

Because I was now three years into my loss, I had accumulated quite a library. Celina had a thirst for answers and would often borrow some of my books. We had great spiritual conversations.

While I was visiting Carol in Mississippi, Celina was visiting her family in India. She called me when she returned to say that she had brought me back a present from India. I was anxious to see what it was.

Celina had bought me a copy of the book *Autobiography of a Yogi*. I had never heard of this book, and I was thrilled to have this treasure from India. This book introduced me to some new concepts of religion, God, and spirituality. These aspects tied in well with what I had been reading about life and death. It also validated my personal experiences with the paranormal and really gave me food for thought. I immediately shared this with Carol in Mississippi.

She wanted to get a copy of the book, but I told her that I wasn't sure that she could get the book here since Celina had purchased it in India. She was going to check one of her bookstores anyway.

A few weeks later, she told me that not only was she able to get the book, but that it was actually on the bookstore's shelves. She didn't even have to order it. I told her that it couldn't be the same book since this book was first printed in 1946, and I really couldn't imagine even an updated version of it being in a small Southern bookstore. She said that it was. Once she described the cover and some more details to me, I knew that it really was the same book.

One day while she was sitting reading the book, Jason came home and asked her, "Where did you get that book from? That's the same book that Geri was pointing to at Graceland and saying how Elvis was a seeker, also."

Carol looked rather startled and told Jason that he must be mistaken, that she didn't remember seeing that book at Graceland. Jason swore it was the same book. Carol still didn't think so.

Later that day, Jason decided to look through the material that he had picked up at Graceland the day we had visited. He walked over to Carol as she was reading her book and said, "Look at this."

Carol said that one of the booklets from Graceland mentioned that Elvis had indeed had a copy of the book. Not only that, he had purchased and given out hundreds of copies of the book. He had also visited the Self-Realization Fellowship in California. Carol was stunned.

I called Celina to discuss the synchronicity of all this, and she added a bit more to the story. She said that the purchase of that book was sort of by accident. She told me that she had missed the bus she was supposed to have taken and ended up in the city with some time on her hands. She decided to browse around in one of the bookstores while she waited for her bus. She said that as she was looking at the book, a thought passed through her mind telling her to buy the book for me.

Of all the books in the world, the one I was pointing to in Mississippi was the same book that Celina was buying for me in India during the same time period. This seemed far beyond the realm of coincidence.

I remembered this account again when I received my 1994 spring catalogue from the A.R.E. Press. On page 11 of that catalogue was the same book that Carol and I now had (thanks to Celina). I just burst out laughing. What a message! I stopped to consider the significant words in the names of the two organizations involved. A.R.E. stands for Association for *Research* and *Enlightenment,* and the Yogi is connected to *self-realization.* Could it be true that our enlightenment really does come from our self-realization— our searching within ourselves? Do we have the necessary components to accomplish our purpose on earth within us now?

The Cayce material stressed the importance of prayer and meditation. Prayer was our talking with God; while meditation was our listening to God. The answer was within us. This is an empowering concept, and I believe that it is a true one.

As I look back, I can see that my vacation trip turned out to be more than just a pleasure trip. I find it very significant that Elvis was used as a symbol in my dream six months before this trip actually took place. Not only did I see some more new dots appearing on my spiritual canvas, I sensed some vague understanding awakening in my brain.

It's interesting to note that Celina does not own a copy of

this book. Yet she felt compelled to buy the book for me. Why? Since she is as desperate in her search for answers as I am, wouldn't it have been more logical for her to have purchased the book for herself and not for me?

If she had done that, though, I would never have been able to make any sense of the Elvis dream with the rest of its message. The information in that book was meant for me to know; that's for sure.

I think that it was through this particular book that I began to get the sense of the universal connection. I had been steadily waking up to the fact that perhaps from birth on things are connected in our own personal lives to bring us through this lifetime. I was focused on just the individual at that point. But, believe me, even that focus was a tremendous accomplishment for my brain, which seemed to have lived on another planet for the past twenty years.

I felt as Columbus might have when he started out on waters that appeared to many to be flat and with edges. Suppose that he really could have fallen off the edge of the earth? Of course, he didn't; but imagine the fear if one believed in that concept.

Well, that was I. As I edged into this ocean of knowledge, don't think that I didn't have my many moments of wondering if I were going to fall off the edge. I didn't, however, and with this realization came a loss of fear and a sense of deep peace. It takes courage to embark on a spiritual journey. But, believe me, it's worth it.

I noticed a sensation of connectedness. I seemed to know that I was connected to everyone on this earth somehow. How, I wasn't sure, but I knew this was a correct assumption.

The fact of geography alone had driven home that point to me. When I considered that I was in Mississippi and Celina had been halfway across the world in India, yet a thought had connected us. That's pretty powerful—connected by a thought, a mere thought. Are our thoughts really that potent?

Perhaps that is why Jesus condemned negative thoughts as much as negative actions. I had never understood this before and actually had thought that it was quite picky on His part to do that. But if this concept of thought having power was correct, I could then see why He would caution this.

Suddenly, the dots on my canvas were not just isolated spots all across the surface, making it look chaotic and messy. There was actually a picture beginning to take form here. I couldn't quite make it out yet, but lines seemed to be starting to connect those dots and actually to be making a pattern.

I would soon acquire the book *Your Life* by Bruce McArthur, and this would eventually help me to fill in the missing lines. Again, it's interesting to note that I did not originally order this book; it was a member selection by A.R.E. Yet it seemed to become a powerful enhancer in my new spiritual picture. I was so impressed by this book that I ordered five copies and gave them to close friends as gifts. I did this because I was noticing that my most influential books were coming to me by people or means that had not been of my own intent. Was the universe teaching me something? Was God guiding me if I would let Him?

Yes, my vacation trip turned out to be a crucial growth point in my new focus. June 9 had become significant for the third time in my life.

14

Others Are Affected

*"Many miracles and wonders were being performed . . .
and more and more became believers."*   Acts 5:12, 14

IN JUNE OF 1991, a large portrait of Heather was finally completed and arrived at our house. The only wall that could really do the portrait justice was the one that Heather's tall bureau was against. We decided to move the bureau to the space where her TV was and to put the TV on top of this tall bureau. We would then use her night stand to hold whatever pictures and memorabilia we could fit on it.

I had finally mustered up enough courage to go through several things in Heather's closet. Some of these items I decided to display on the night stand with her special pictures and yearbook. Two of these items were stickers. The larger one was the "Body Glove" emblem and had been one of Heather's favorite symbols. She had used this symbol as part of the design she had created for her cousin Mike's jacket.

The smaller sticker was a surfing symbol of "Hang Ten." Although Heather had never surfed, she had intended to learn as soon as she had finished her treatments and was back on her feet again. She was an excellent water-skier, and Mike (who was a surfer) had promised to teach her to surf as soon as she was ready. So this sticker served as a symbol of a future dream for her.

I did not know that she had these stickers until I went through some of the boxes in her closet. Since these were the only stickers in her possession and I knew how symbolic they were for her, I decided to display them with her other precious items. Therefore, when we selected items to be placed on the night stand next to this new portrait, these two stickers became a part of this new display.

About a week after this portrait arrived in our home, Mike called to tell us that he had returned from Florida and would be here for the summer to help run the family business. We had not seen him since the funeral. We were anxious to visit with him and to have him view Heather's new portrait. We also planned to share the "calla-lily incident" with him to see what he thought about it.

It was so nice to see him. Yet, as I watched him arrive in his red jeep, I couldn't help but remember his teaching Heather how to drive his jeep a few weeks before she died. I could picture the two of them laughing as he tried to teach her how to shift in our driveway. It was a bittersweet memory.

Now, Mike sat alone as he drove into our driveway. A sad look crossed his young, handsome face. He cried as he held us. We finally walked into the house and began chatting and catching up on what had been happening over the long winter months. I told him about my secret research, my doubts about my religion, and the "calla-lily incident."

Mike did not seem to have a problem understanding this strange event. He told us that he often sensed Heather's presence in Florida and even at times when he was surfing. He then asked me if he could see her new portrait. He also wanted us to demonstrate the movement of the pictures in her bedroom on that special night of her prom anniversary.

Walt, Mike, and I walked into her bedroom. I was explaining to him that we had moved the bureau to accommodate this new picture and that I had to put some of the items onto the night stand that had originally been on her bureau. I was not looking at Mike at that second. Suddenly I heard Walt say to Mike, "What's the matter?"

I turned to look at Mike's face and saw that he was wide-eyed and speechless. He kept pointing at Heather's night stand and trying to say something to us. I asked him what was wrong.

He grabbed both Walt and me by the hand and began to pull us out of the room. He kept saying, "You just won't believe this; come and see!"

Suddenly, he had us outside and next to his red jeep. I anxiously replied, "What?" I had no idea what we were all supposed to be looking at.

He stammered, "Look!" as he pointed to the rims of his tires on the jeep. I looked down at the right wheel and saw the "Body Glove" sticker in the middle of the wheel rim.

He grabbed my hand again and led me to the left side of the jeep. As he pointed, I observed the "Hang Ten" sticker in the middle of the wheel rim. They were the same stickers (one being larger than the other) that were on Heather's night stand. They were an identical match.

At this time, I still only knew to use the word *coincidence* to describe this phenomenon. And this word I voiced aloud. The three of us stood speechless for a few minutes, awed by this symbolic connection.

Mike explained to us that he had changed his tires approximately a week before in preparation for driving back home for the summer. He told us the thought had crossed his mind that the rims of his wheels just looked "plain," and so he had put some stickers on them to brighten them up a bit.

He told us that as he looked through a bag that contained about a hundred stickers, he tried to decide if he wanted the two sides to be the same or different. He told us that he just felt that he should have two different stickers, and these were the two that he had picked.

I had not talked to Mike in over a month and I knew that he did not know about my two stickers on the night stand. I also had not spoken with my cousin Pat (Mike's mother) in over a week. Since my cousin runs a summer business, she had been very busy getting things in order and had not even had a chance to come by to see Heather's new portrait.

The few people who had seen Heather's new picture hardly knew Mike. So, there was really no way that Mike could have even subconsciously been aware of my sticker display.

Since it was early in my search at that point and I was not yet aware of synchronicity, I viewed this as simply being extremely coincidental for at least another year or so.

With the "calla-lily incident" I had started to open up to people and to share some of my research, my doubts, my feelings, and my unique experiences, but I was also beginning to really listen more to other people's experiences.

For almost twenty years of my life I had talked at people to try to proselytize them. Now, it seemed like my listening skills had really become super-sharpened, and I was becoming aware that I was not the only person to have experienced some form of unique phenomenon in my life.

People suddenly began to share their intimate accounts with me. They seemed to tell me things sometimes without my even asking them. The difference was that I was truly listening for the first time in almost twenty years.

The first person to tell me something unique was my mother. She told me that she had tried to tell me about this before but that I would not listen. Instead I would attempt to preach to her; so she just gave up trying. When she finally confided in me, it was actually to reassure me that Walt and I were not losing our minds.

I had gotten brave enough to tell her about some of the incidents that were happening in my life at that time. One of the events I first shared with her took place one night after I had a vivid dream of an encounter with one of my elders.

In the dream, the elder was threatening me, telling me that Kim would die with me if I were to leave the religious organization. (This was still the time of my secret research.) I was furious with him, but I was also very frightened. The dream became so intense that I woke myself up.

As I came awake, my heart pounding and my breathing heavy, I came face to face with my father. Oddly enough, it was only his face. It was larger than his real face, and there was no body or form visible; but it was his face. I was positively awake. He didn't say anything. He just kept looking at me. I whispered, "Daddy?"

As soon as I verbalized this, his face began to rotate slowly in a clockwise manner and began to move backward and away from me. But a most startling thing suddenly happened. This rotation seemed to produce more hair on his head, and when the rotation stopped for a second, the face became Heather's face.

I sat up and called, "Heather?" She looked at me for a second and then seemed to quickly rotate backward out of my bedroom door.

Walt woke up and asked me what had happened. I explained to him about the face. Neither of us could think of an explanation for this phenomenon. It had never happened to me before and (to this day) has never happened to me again. Yet I am positive that I was awake.

When I finally shared this with my mother, she didn't seem at all surprised. She confided in me about her experience. She told me that several years ago she had gone to visit my father's sister, my Aunt Virginia. As she was lying there trying to fall asleep, she began to notice some movement in the corner of the room.

She said that something like a whirling cloud seemed to be moving toward her. Suddenly, she could see my father as clear as day. She reached out to touch him but could not seem to reach that far. She sat up in bed and said, "My God, it's Joe!"

She told me that as soon as she said these words aloud, she could hear a "whooshing" sound and that he just seemed to move rapidly away from her. I asked her if she could have been dreaming. She said, "Positively no." She was awake.

She shared this experience with my aunt and uncle the next morning. They did not seem to have a problem believing that it was my father. It seemed that everyone (except me) had no problem believing things of this sort, even in those days.

Again, she explained that she had tried to share this with me years before, but I was not receptive to it at all. She said that, since my preaching at her intimidated her, she thought that she best keep this experience to herself. I was greatly comforted by her sharing this with me now.

Since people were really opening up to me, I began to record these different accounts over the next few years. I did this so that I would remember these fascinating experiences. I didn't realize that there was a common thread involved here. I had no idea then that these experiences would prove to be very healing for me and would eventually become part of this book. I have included a few of these experiences in this chapter in order to demonstrate that I am not alone in this journey.

PAT'S ACCOUNT: My cousin Pat had an interesting experience a few months after my encounter with the sequins.

One day as she was cleaning in her basement, she suddenly noticed a sparkling blue sequin on her basement floor. She wondered how it could have gotten there.

She had helped Heather work on her prom gown two years before, but that had been upstairs in her sewing room. Heather's gown had never been downstairs. Since Pat's dogs stay downstairs most of the time (and shed), she vacuums this area almost daily. She was puzzled.

She said she bent over to pick up the sequin and felt a wave of nostalgia come over her. She went to sit on the couch for a minute and noticed that Mike had left some of his things on the couch since he had just returned home from Florida again. She was annoyed at first and went to move some of them. The first thing that she picked up was Mike's jacket.

As she picked up the jacket, the "Body Glove" symbol suddenly faced her. She remembered how hard Heather had worked on Mike's jacket and how many compliments he had received for Heather's work. Pat held the jacket close to her and started to cry. She swore that she felt Heather's presence at that time.

Interestingly, Mike had not been home for Heather's prom, nor did he have any of Heather's prom gown sequins in his possession. So there was really no logical reason as to how the sequin got there. But what moved Pat the most was the connection of the sequin with Mike's just arriving home and leaving his favorite jacket on the couch. She feels that Heather's presence was there on that day.

THE PENNY ACCOUNT: The summer of the Memphis experience I was in Heather's room one day and found a penny in the middle of the room. Heather had left a penny on her night stand and, since I saw no reason to ever remove it, it had remained there.

I looked over at the night stand and realized that the penny was missing, and I assumed that someone (maybe one of the smaller children) had picked it up and then dropped it. I really didn't think too much about this and placed it back on the stand.

Later that night, Kathy and Kevin came over and were planning to spend the night. Kathy and I went into Heather's room to put the overnight bags in there. While Kathy and I were in the room, I told her about the penny in the middle of the room. We discussed the various meanings that this penny could have.

Since the penny had no real significant meaning to me at the time, I did not connect it with Heather at all. Kathy, however, happened to remember the movie *Ghost* and the movement of the penny in that movie. She wondered if it were possible that Heather was trying to tell us something with this penny.

We really didn't have any basis for thinking this, so I jokingly mentioned to Kathy that since I had been reading and thinking so much lately, perhaps the penny meant "A penny for your thoughts." Kathy suggested that it could be due to the words, "In God We Trust." I said, "Good thought."

We went back into the kitchen with Walt and Kevin. We had decided not to tell them about the penny incident. Since Kevin has almost visionlike dreams of Heather (in which he can ask her questions and receive answers), we decided we would wait to see if anything would happen during the night since they would be sleeping in her room.

Walt and I retired upstairs to our room at about 11:00 p.m. Kathy and Kevin were very anxious and couldn't sleep. They watched TV for a while and talked. They tried to sleep, but were distracted by every little noise. When morning came, they were very disappointed that nothing had happened during the night. After breakfast, they returned home.

Kathy awoke the next morning and noticed that Kevin was not in bed. Instantly, she knew that he had made contact with Heather that night. She ran downstairs to find him writing in his journal.

He told her that he had dreamed about Heather that night. As Kevin related the dream, he remarked that one thing that Heather had said to him did not seem to make any sense at all in the context of the dream.

Kathy asked him what it was that didn't make sense. He looked at Kathy and said, "Well, she said something about a penny; she said that it wasn't a penny for your thoughts; it's a penny from heaven." He went on to explain that Heather had told him to tell this to Aunt Geri (me), but he said that this seemed rather silly to him.

He barely got the words out of his mouth when Kathy's face went white. When Kevin asked her what was the matter, she repeated to him the conversation that she and I had had about the penny on the day before. Kevin was very shocked.

But that didn't end it. Two days later, Kathy went into her family room and found two pennies in front of Heather's picture, and the picture had been turned sideways. Kathy and Kevin had no idea where those pennies had come from nor how they had gotten where they were. Also, Kathy remarked that since they were face up, it was a reminder that "In God We Trust."

Months later, I was reading an article about Bernie Siegel in *New Age Journal,* in which it mentioned that he kept finding pennies with their message "In God We Trust." I burst out laughing and immediately recalled my experience with the penny as well as Kathy and Kevin's experience.

I called Kathy. We both felt strengthened by the article and knew that this was further verification that we were indeed on the right track. Trust in God's wisdom and "go with the flow" were the penny's new symbols for us.

Kevin has serious back problems. As a result, he went on pain medication shortly after the penny experience. It's interesting to note that once Kevin was put on pain medication, he was not able to have the visionlike dreams of Heather.

When he is not on medication, he sometimes has them;

when he is on medication, the effect of it seems to interfere with this type of experience. We are not sure why this is so, but Kevin has kept records. The medication definitely stops the experience for him.

Just before Kevin went on pain medication, Kathy walked downstairs one morning to find two pictures of Heather moved from their original positions. She put them back in place. She asked me what it could mean, but I had no concrete answer.

The next morning, Kevin woke Kathy up at 6:00 a.m. and told her that Heather had contacted him once again that night in a visionlike dream. In the vision, Heather told him that she had been leaving signs for them. She also told him that their beloved shepherd dog, King, was with her now and that he liked her.

This fact amazed Kathy because King had never liked Heather. When she visited Kathy and Kevin, Heather had always teased King, who was kept on a chain. Hence, King was not overly fond of Heather, to say the least.

Kathy quickly got out of bed and went downstairs into the family room. Immediately, she noticed that the 5" x 7" picture of Heather was completely turned sideways. Another smaller picture of Heather had also been moved.

What probably affected Kathy the most was that a small picture of King had been moved four pictures up and was also facing sideways. Right next to it was the sideways picture of Heather. As Kathy puts it, "They were face to face!"

She felt that this was proof to her that King was really with Heather. She had so lamented King's death (a month before) and wondered what had happened to him. She now felt at peace over this new revelation.

CELINA AND DON'S ACCOUNT: Celina's husband, Don, is gifted with the ability to see visions. He frequently sees and communicates with their deceased daughter, Malini.

One day, when I went to their house to have lunch, I brought Celina a bouquet of flowers to bring to Malini's grave. We spent the whole afternoon talking about our deceased children. Don was not at home, so Celina filled him in on our visit.

That night Don had a vision of Malini, and she brought another girl, a teenager, with her. Don had never been in our house and had never seen a picture of Heather. Since he did not know the girl with Malini, he asked Celina if she could get a picture from me so that he could see if it was Heather.

I gave Celina a copy of the picture we had used for Heather's gravestone. It was one of the last pictures we had taken of her before she lost her hair from the chemotherapy.

Don looked at the picture and said that, although the face and eyes and features were the same as the girl in the vision, it must not be Heather because the girl he saw had straight hair and it was more brown than blond, like the picture indicated. Celina was so disappointed, since she had hoped that our children were friends on the other side.

She was in for a pleasant surprise, however. I explained to Celina that Heather did indeed have straight brown hair. The photo I had given to Celina was part of Heather's senior picture portfolio, and she had gotten a spiral perm several months before these pictures were taken. She had also had blond highlights put in so that her hair looked more blond than brown in this particular picture.

Celina was thrilled. So were Don, Walt, and I. We believe that our friendship was not by accident and that our children are alive and are friends on the other side. This brings all of us comfort.

ELWOOD'S ACCOUNT: Elwood and Cynthia had planned to tour Alaska during August of 1993. Approximately a week before they left, I had a disturbing dream about them. In the dream, I saw rooms full of people moving about and talking. The mood seemed very sad. Suddenly, Elwood was before me and he was crying.

I seemed very uncomfortable with him crying because he has always been such a strong and stable friend and always appears to be very much in control. Yet, in this dream, he seemed so deep into his grief.

I came awake very sad and somewhat anxious. I wondered if Jennifer, who has been chronically ill since birth, was OK. I wondered, too, why in the dream Cynthia seemed more in control, and this would be out of character for her to be more so than Elwood.

I recorded the dream in my journal and told their daughter, Heather, about the dream. I asked her if Jennifer was all right, as well as the rest of the family members. Heather assured me that everything was fine. I still felt uneasy about their upcoming trip. I shared this dream with several of our other friends. I did not, however, mention this to Elwood or Cynthia.

I called Heather frequently while they were away to check on Jennifer. Everything was going fine. A week before they were scheduled to return, Heather called and told me that Elwood's mother had fallen and would require hip surgery. I felt somewhat anxious, but again she assured me that things would be OK.

A few days later, things were no longer fine. Complications arose and we became concerned about her survival. Elwood and Cynthia were notified in Alaska.

Elwood told me that a few days before they were scheduled to come home, a strange thing happened to him. On this day, they were having breakfast on a boat. He told me that during most of their breakfast time, things were relatively quiet since no music was playing at the time.

Suddenly, music began to play. The music seemed to draw their attention. Their friends and the other people in the restaurant began to look around and say, "What's with this music?"

Elwood told me that the music seemed to be from something out of the 1930s—music that you would associate with death or dying. He said that it was not scary music; it was more of a sad, but peaceful death scene.

As that thought passed through his mind, an odd feeling of warmth and peace went through him. He said that he instantly knew that his mother had just died.

As soon as they could get off the boat, Elwood told Cynthia that he needed to make a phone call. He did not want to upset the friends whom they were traveling with, so he waited until he and Cynthia were on their way to the phone booth before he told Cynthia that he knew that his mother had just died.

Elwood called the hospital in Rhode Island. His instinct was sadly correct. His mother had died in Rhode Island at the same time that he had heard the song and had had the feeling in Alaska.

When Heather called to tell us about her grandmother, we now understood the meaning of my dream. Elwood was shown to be more affected in the dream because it was his mother who had died. The connection was more to him as an individual than to them as a couple (as it would have been if it were one of their children).

Many people had known about the dream and were anxiously awaiting Elwood and Cynthia's return. As I stated, we had not shared this with either Cynthia or Elwood before they left since we did not want to put a damper on their vacation.

After Elwood told us about his experience in Alaska, we confided in him about the dream. He was amazed to learn this fact and was glad that he did not know this before he left on vacation. He does believe that his mother came to him in Alaska to say goodbye. He also felt that she was letting him know that she was at peace on the other side and was still with him.

Elwood confided in Walt and me that his mother's death

was easier for him to accept because of all that we had experienced since Heather's death. He felt that Heather was not only a teaching instrument for Walt and me, but also for his family and our other friends. I, too, believe this to be true.

DOMENIC'S ACCOUNT: Dom had been a student of mine some ten years earlier, and he had managed to gain a very special place in my heart. After graduation from high school, Dom was promoted to be the manager of one of the sections in a large grocery store near us. Since I shopped at this store, he would frequently see Heather and me while we were in the store.

Heather got a part-time job in the store during her junior year in high school. She held this job until her condition prevented her from working steadily. Dom was devastated when he learned about Heather's condition. So was everyone else in that store. They were wonderful to her and very kind and supportive.

Heather had given Dom a picture of herself, which he carried around with him constantly. Coincidentally, his mother-in-law also developed cancer during the same time period as Heather did. Both of them died in 1990, Heather in September and his mother-in-law in December. Dom was crushed. He had loved them both.

To make this situation even more unsettling, Dom developed cancer in 1992. I was stunned and saddened. Dom had taken a job out of state and I had not seen him much since Heather's death.

When he called in the spring of 1993 to tell me about his condition, he sounded very upbeat on the phone. He showed more concern for me in coping with Heather's death than he did for his own condition. I was touched by this, but I urged him to read books such as *Love, Medicine, and Miracles.* I urged him to meditate and to try to stay focused.

I didn't hear from him again for almost a year. I was getting to the point of panicking and was going to try to get in touch with him through his father. I began to think that something was wrong.

Just about that time, he called to tell me that I had been heavy on his mind, and he wanted to arrange to come and visit with me the next time that he was in town. I was thrilled! He had no idea that I had left my religious organization and was now in the process of writing a book.

I was a little nervous about telling him about my encounters with Heather. I had been his accounting teacher in high school, and he remembered me as being pretty strict in my religion. So I wondered how he would react to all of this.

Actually, he was more amazed by the religious structure and how and why I left than he was about the other experiences. When I asked him why, he said, "Although I don't tell too many people this, I've had some unusual things happen to me, too."

He proceeded to tell me that Heather's picture and his deceased mother-in-law's picture are always on his bureau. He told me that they are a constant source of strength and courage for him. He had so admired the bravery of these two special people in their battle with cancer. He said that they were a constant inspiration to him. Just knowing how he felt about Heather strengthened the bond between us.

He proceeded to explain to me that because of this inspiration, he felt confident in his battle—except for a brief time. He told me that during that time, he had come to Rhode Island to visit his family and was staying with his sister. His sister had purchased his deceased grandmother's home and was now living in it. Dom had been given his grand-mother's car.

He told me that one evening he had walked out to the car to get something. Suddenly he heard his grandmother's voice say, "Nani's little boy." He was startled. He looked around, but no one was there. He got what he needed from the car and went back inside.

His mother was there, and he told her what he thought he had heard. She started to cry and told him that his grandmother had always called him that. He told me that his whole family felt comfortable with the concept of his grandmother being still able to communicate with them. He just added, "We don't tell too many people this."

He proceeded to explain to me that later, on that same night, he was sitting on his bed and preparing to meditate before retiring for the evening. He told me that something in the corner of the room caught his eye. He glanced up to see his grandmother standing there, looking at him. When she caught his eye, she waved and smiled at him. She then began walking out of the room and down the hall to her old bedroom.

I asked him if she said anything to him verbally or by mental communication. He said, "No." I asked him if she appeared as a form or dressed as a person. He told me that she was as he remembered her except that she looked as if someone had lightly erased her features.

He was positive that it was his grandmother. I asked him if she walked through the wall, and he told me that she had gone out the doorway and down the hall. He told me that after she did this, a peaceful feeling came over him.

The next morning, when he woke up, he knew that he was going to be OK. He thought that she had come to convey this message to him and that it was not his time yet.

Dom has been in remission since August 1993. He became so assured about this that he began to do meditations and imagery. He also told his doctor that he would not lose his hair though his doctor told him he would. Dom did not lose his hair, and he is still as handsome as ever.

He credits Heather and his mother-in-law as the inspiration to believe that he could win this battle. He believes that they, as well as his grandmother, helped him through this time period. I believe this, also. My thoughts and prayers stay with him that he remain in remission.

GINNY'S ACCOUNT: Exactly one year after we buried Heather, Ginny's mother died. September 28 now means as much to Ginny as it does to us. The *Daily Word* with which I start my day is a gift from Ginny in memory of her mother.

Shortly after her mother died, Ginny came to understand the significance of the butterfly to her mother. As the calla lily is to me a symbol of Heather, the butterfly became Ginny's symbol of her mother. Ginny eventually designed and knitted me a gorgeous sweater with both a calla lily and a butterfly on it. I had not been aware of the symbol of the butterfly before her mother's death, since Ginny herself had not yet realized its significance.

Although Ginny's mother died in Florida, her memorial service to commemorate the burial of the ashes was held a month later in Massachusetts. With this event, we would soon become aware of the connection of the butterfly with Ginny's mother. The day of the memorial service, the minister in charge had printed up programs to be distributed before the service. The cover, a butterfly, did not yet mean anything to me, but I assumed that Ginny had selected this since she had put the program together. However, I learned something quite different.

As Ginny explained to me days later, she had been standing at the graveside listening to the minister when she noticed a white butterfly flying around. She told me that she remembers thinking how unusual it was for a butterfly to still be out in late October. She also told me that the minister had picked out the cover for the program but for no particular reason that she knew about. At this time, she made no conscious connection between the two events.

A few days later, Ginny began going through her mother's personal things. She suddenly realized the number of times she found butterfly items and symbols amongst her mother's belongings. As these thoughts came to her mind, she then reflected back to the white butterfly at her mother's grave site and the minister coincidentally having already chosen the butterfly for the program cover. The butterfly rapidly emerged as a symbol for her mother, a symbol that Ginny had not been aware of before. This symbol, however, would consistently reinforce itself in the future.

Therefore, since 1991, the butterfly has been an instant representation of Ginny's mother. One day after her father became ill, I was walking along the road when suddenly a beautiful black butterfly with blue spots fringed in white landed near the white line of the break-down lane and a few feet from where I happened to be walking.

Immediately I thought of Ginny's mother. I began to feel a bit anxious about Ginny's father. It is very odd for a butterfly to just land on a fairly busy, well-traveled road.

When I came in from my walk, I found a call from Ginny on my answering machine. I returned her call and told her about the butterfly. This was Wednesday, July 6, 1994. I knew that she was leaving to go back to Florida on Friday, July 8. I assumed that she had called me to say goodbye.

Sadly she had other news to relate. She told me that her father was being transferred to a hospice hospital the next day and probably had only about a month to live. We reflected on the fact that she had been back home for about a month now and that she had purchased her ticket for Friday a month ago. She also told me that she felt that she would not see her father alive again and that she had said a quiet goodbye to him when she had left him last month.

But, over the last month, he seemed to be coming around and she began to think that maybe he would recover from the surgery after all. Her dad kept telling the rest of the family that he wanted to go home. Ginny and I had wondered what he meant by home—his house or heaven with her mom.

We talked about many things, but especially the significance of the butterfly that day. Perhaps her mother was around for a reason. Ginny was glad that she had purchased her ticket a month before and would be leaving to see her father on Friday. I told her that I would call her in Florida in a few days.

Friday morning, Ginny called me at 7:30 a.m. with the sad news. Her father had died in the night. Since it was after midnight, it was Friday, July 8. (Coincidentally, that is my father's birthday.) How strange that she had picked the exact date for her ticket. If she hadn't already purchased her ticket a month before, she would have been trying to book a flight for that day anyway.

As she had previously told me, she had secretly said goodbye to her father a month before. She had felt then that she would never see him alive again. Yes, he wanted to go home. But home to him just could have been heaven.

The butterfly was quite a coincidence. I had never seen a butterfly land on this busy road in the years that I have been walking this route. It's interesting, too, that it would happen after Ginny got the news that her father probably had only a month left to live. And it would happen the day before he died, on my father's birthday.

CINDY AND MIKE'S ACCOUNT: In my early years of teaching at Chariho, we employed a secretary named Cindy. Cindy eventually was offered another job and left our school system. I had not seen her in more than ten years when Heather died.

Cindy and Mike had lost their son, Patrick, in November of 1984. Patrick had been hit by a car while riding his bike to the bus stop. A sad fact would tie Patrick and Heather together. Patrick died a day-and-a-half after his accident in the same hospital and the same pediatric intensive care ward that Heather would die in six years later. Obviously, we did not know this then.

Cindy and Mike were well aware of the intense grief that parents suffer over the loss of a child. They spoke with friends of ours and wanted us to know that they were there for us if we needed them. It was almost a year before we felt able to talk to another couple who had lost a child.

Cindy and Mike were wonderful. Although I had never met Mike before and Walt did not know either of them, we immediately felt a sadly unique bond with them. We became very comfortable with them and, during the course of the evening, we began to tell them about the "calla-lily incident."

They did not seem to find this surprising nor unusual. Cindy sensed that I was not comfortable with our experiences because of the formal religious structure that I was still involved with. She tried to ease my fear by volunteering to share some of their experiences with us.

As she began, she did say that they don't tell these experiences to everyone because of the strange looks that people will sometimes give them. She did point out, however, that parents who lose children seem to always be receptive and comforted by knowing that they are not alone with their unique experiences. Walt and I were tremendously reassured and comforted by knowing that we were not alone on our journey, nor were we crazy.

Cindy and Mike are practicing Catholics. They have always believed that experiences of this nature enhance their religious experience rather than contradict it, as I had been taught to believe.

Cindy then proceeded to relate to us that she and Mike shared a unique experience simultaneously hours before Patrick officially died. Cindy had been trying to get a few hours' sleep in the intensive care waiting room (the same room where I, too, had tried to sleep), while Mike sat out his watch over Patrick.

Patrick was in a coma with severe head injuries. He was scheduled to have a brain-wave test in the morning to see if his condition had improved since the time of his accident the morning before. Cindy had not slept since the previous night and was trying to get a few hours' sleep before changing places with Mike. Yet she could not seem to sleep.

Around 1:30 a.m., she was compelled to go in with Mike and Patrick. She told me that as soon as she approached Patrick's bed, she felt an overwhelming sense of emptiness. She pointed out that there wasn't any change in any of the machines that were attached to Patrick, yet she just knew inside of herself that Patrick's spirit had left his body.

Before she could verbalize this thought to Mike, she heard Mike say, "He's gone; I felt him leave." She then conveyed to Mike her thoughts and her feelings of emptiness. They both knew then what the brain test would reveal in the morning. They also made their decision regarding Patrick remaining on the respirator or not.

After completing the morning testing, the doctors told Mike and Cindy what they already knew to be true. The tests showed no brain activity, and Mike and Cindy were informed that Patrick would not survive. The decision to disconnect Patrick from the respirator would be left to Mike and Cindy.

Around 7:30 p.m. of November 8, 1984, Patrick was disconnected from the respirator and died within the minute. The hole left inside of Mike and Cindy's hearts has still not healed over these last ten years; and, as Cindy says, "It won't until the day we die."

Although Mike and Cindy instinctively (and simultaneously) knew that Patrick had left his body at 1:30 a.m., something would happen to them to indicate that God had confirmed this for them. A remarkable sign was about to be given to them.

Cindy went to bed at about 10:00 p.m. that night. She said that, oddly enough, she fell into a very deep sleep for about four hours. When she awoke, she felt a need to go into Patrick's room and lie in his bed and hold his pillow. Since Patrick's brother, Matthew, shared the room with him, Cindy tried to be very quiet so as not to disturb him.

She was lying in Patrick's bed for what she feels was close to an hour. She said that she slowly became aware of a red flashing light and realized that she was staring at Patrick's alarm clock. What she was beginning to notice was that the alarm clock was flashing "1:30" over and over again, even though it was near 3:00 a.m.

At first she thought that there had been a power failure and that was why the clock was flashing. Yet, she wondered why it wasn't flashing the standard "12:00" that all the old digitals always flashed after a power failure.

As she moved in Patrick's bed, Matthew woke up. She comforted him and pointed out the clock to him. Matthew told her that no one else had been in Patrick's room that day and to reach the cord to this clock would involve actually moving furniture. In other words, it could not have been disconnected by accident. And why was 1:30, the time they felt Patrick had died, flashing? The other clocks in the house displayed the correct time; therefore, there couldn't have been a power failure.

Since it was now after midnight, officially it was November 9, Cindy's fortieth birthday. She said that she feels, even today, that Patrick was present and was trying to tell her that he was with them. Perhaps this was a gift from God for her fortieth birthday.

Cindy has always been strong in her faith. She said that she never doubted for a minute that Patrick was in heaven with God as an angel. She always believed that he was fine and happy with God. It was she and Mike who obviously were the ones in pain now.

I truly envied her faith at that moment. I was stunned by her firm conviction. Why had I not felt like that when Heather died? Why had Cindy and Mike shown up in our lives at exactly this time?

It was during this period that we both found out that our children had died not only in the same hospital but also in the same ward. We both live in an area where we are within a half to three-quarters of an hour's ride to some fine hospitals. An hour to an hour-and-a-half adds some other larger and well-known medical facilities. What was the chance that they would die in almost the same bed, in the same hospital, and in the same pediatric unit (given that Heather was a cancer patient just five weeks shy of her eighteenth birthday and Patrick was a young accident victim)? I really felt some connection here.

Cindy and Mike were an essential aid at this time in my life. Because they were not emotionally involved with us at the time of Heather's death, nor at the time of the "calla-lily incident," they represented to me an objective and impartial source of validating my experiences so far.

The coincidence of our children dying in the same place immediately made me sit up and take notice. The fact that she had shared a unique experience with me and felt it validated religion instead of destroying it also drew my attention.

Although I had not at that time officially resigned from my religious organization, in my heart I knew it was coming. Having Cindy and Mike enter our lives at this time and with the information they possessed seemed to affirm something within myself.

I pressed Cindy further to see if she had experienced dreams or the feeling of Patrick's presence after that initial night. She decided to share something else with us.

She explained that, approximately three weeks after Patrick died, Mike had urged her to come with him to a Christmas bazaar for Patrick's school. Although she really did not feel like going out in public, she said she had a strong urge to go.

She said that she and Mike had always wanted a manger for their home. As they walked around the bazaar, they suddenly came upon one of the most beautiful mangers they had ever seen. The bid was to start at $190, and she felt that they really did not have the extra money at that time. Mike bid anyway.

They were informed that a woman from out of town kept

calling in to place a bid, and Cindy felt that they probably would not get this manger. As she walked past the kitchen, she saw her son Michael talking on the phone. She heard him making bids up to $325 and quickly signaled him, "No!" Too late; his bid had won.

Michael and two other women had made a combined pledge of $100 toward it as a gift for Cindy and Mike. Her son knew how much his parents had wanted this particular manger. As Cindy said, "It really was the most beautiful manger I had ever seen in my life."

What the women confided in Cindy was even more interesting. They told her that they had been working on the figurines for this manger and praying the rosary for Patrick on the day that he died.

One of the women was having difficulty painting the face of the Baby Jesus. She had tried to paint it several times. On the day of Patrick's accident, she began again while praying for Patrick. She was able to complete the face that day. So, when they saw Cindy and Mike at the bazaar and realized their interest in the manger, they couldn't help but connect this project to the "blood, sweat, and tears" put into this for Patrick. They especially wanted Cindy and Mike to have it and, hence, they donated the extra money.

Cindy told me that a week later the nun from Patrick's school called to ask her if she had noticed that the "angel of the Lord" was missing from their manger. Cindy said, "I know, we have our own angel, Patrick."

Since Patrick knew that they had always wanted a manger, she considers it a heavenly gift from him for Christmas. She didn't seem to be having difficulty discerning the synchronicity of events even though she, too, was unaware of the word for the process.

I tried to explain my difficulty at this time in tying in events and dreams and wondering which seemed more valid or true. She told me that she thought they all tied in together and are all true and valid. I asked her about dreams and told her some of mine about Heather, especially the one I had on the day that Heather was buried.

She related to me a dream that Mike had of Patrick in which she felt divine guidance was given. She explained that at the time of Patrick's death she was not totally satisfied with her job position, though she really was not unhappy there. She said that one day she received a call at work offering her a position with another company.

Since she had not applied for another job and was totally unaware of this one, she was curious as to why she would receive the offer. She was not interested, even though the salary was higher and the job description seemed enticing. She tried to tactfully refuse, but the woman urged her to take a day to think about it. She talked to Mike about the job, but he told her that it was really up to her. She went to church and said a prayer and contemplated about it. She felt that she should refuse it. Since she felt good about this decision, she believed that she had gotten the correct answer.

Cindy called the woman back the next day and refused the position. Toward the end of the day, the woman called back and offered her more money and more vacation time. The woman asked Cindy to take another day to decide.

She called Mike at work, and again he told her that it was her decision. Cindy felt confused.

The next morning before she left for work, she asked Mike one more time, "What am I going to do?" Since she meant this more as a remark in passing and not as a serious question, she was surprised when she heard Mike say, "You really don't want me to tell you, do you?"

Cindy asked Mike what he meant by that question. Mike told her that he had been awake most of the night because he had experienced an intense dream of Patrick.

In the dream, Patrick told him, "Look, I got this job offer for Mom and she turned it down. How many times does she expect me to go back and ask?"

Patrick also explained to Mike that Cindy had misinterpreted the meaning while she was in church. The job was meant for Cindy and she should take it.

Cindy then realized that whatever meaning she thought she had gotten at church was not the meaning intended from above. She went to work, called the woman, and took the job.

As she explained to me, not only did the work turn out to be fantastic, but it trained her for future advancement in the job position that she now holds. She said that she could not help but think of a card that Patrick had made for their anniversary before he died. It said, "You will always have my love, even when it comes from above."

Originally, she thought that Patrick had written this in order to make it rhyme. But as this thought came rushing through her mind, she began to think that perhaps he knew that he would not be around long and that from above he would guide them.

Without our asking and without Cindy's knowing, she was validating some of our experiences. Dreams of the departed, objects being moved (or changed), a card from a child with a hidden message, synchronistic events, and the same hospital were all things that I had no way of knowing that we shared with Cindy and Mike—and she had no way of knowing about our experiences. Most important, why did they feel the urge to contact us through our friends and offer us assistance. No one else had done this, so far, in my journey. Were they, in a sense, sent by God with a message?

I was so grateful for Cindy and Mike's sharing with us at this particular time in our lives. We had thought that only our close friends or relatives could relate to us, but here we were, realizing that even strangers are connected by a common bond and can be used as God's messengers. True, I was still so new in my spiritual journey that I wasn't sure what was happening. But a personal experience of this caliber was just what was needed at the time.

When I asked Cindy if she ever felt Patrick's presence now,

she gave me an interesting answer. She told me she felt that, as the years went by and as she and Mike became more and more adjusted, Patrick's presence withdrew. She told me that she felt Patrick was more involved with God's work now, and he knew that she and Mike would be OK. Yes, they still have their moments, but, as Cindy says, "They aren't as often any more."

AUNT GRACE'S AND AUNT CARMELLA'S ACCOUNTS: As this chapter neared completion, my Aunt Grace and Aunt Carmella (two of my father's sisters) shared their experiences with me. The amazing thing is that I had never told them I was writing another book, and, of course, they would have had no idea as to its content.

My Aunt Grace had been in Florida all winter, and I had not communicated with her during that time. My Aunt Carmella had been ill over the winter, and I had not shared with her what I was doing.

We had been invited to a family picnic in July. The first person to see us as we arrived just happened to be Aunt Grace. The first words out of her mouth were, "I had a dream about you last night." I laughed and said, "Well, maybe it's because you knew you would be seeing me today."

She smiled at me and said, "When are you going to write another book?" I was stunned. Walt looked at me (so did the friends who were with us, Charlie and Shelia) as I stammered out, "Actually, I have one in progress."

Again she smiled at me and said, "Well, you will have to tell me all about it when I return." (She was going for a walk with a friend and had stopped to greet us as we arrived.)

It was after dinner when Aunt Grace finally asked me again about my book. I was sitting with her and Aunt Carmella when she brought this topic up. Aunt Carmella was immediately interested and she, too, asked me what the book was about.

As I discussed my book, I shared Walt's and my story of

the "calla-lily incident" with them for the first time. Suddenly, Aunt Grace piped up and said, "Oh, Geri, I know that things like that are true."

I was rather startled to hear her agree so quickly. Aunt Grace then continued with a very interesting account of her own that had happened just a few weeks before.

She had recently moved into a new apartment due to some health problems, and she was very unhappy over this move. She said that she was in her bedroom one day looking for something when she noticed a cloud or bright light formation in the corner of her room.

Suddenly out of the cloud formation came her parents (my grandparents) and one of her aunts. She said that her father told her that everything would be OK. She said that she was not frightened by this, but just felt very peaceful. She told me that they stepped backward, waved, and then left.

Aunt Grace then smiled at me and whispered, "I don't tell too many people about this." I was so glad that she had chosen to tell me. I couldn't help but reflect on the timing of this conversation.

To add to this, I thought perhaps my other aunt would be uncomfortable with her sister telling me something of this nature. Instead, to my surprise, I noticed that she was really listening and nodding her head in agreement.

Aunt Carmella was then past her eighty-first birthday. She is considered religious and quite strong in her faith. Therefore, I was hoping that this would not be unsettling for them or contradictory to what they had been reared to believe.

Aunt Carmella then shared with me an experience that had happened to her over the past winter. She had been very ill. One night she awoke to see her deceased husband, my Uncle Frank, standing near her bed. She described what he was wearing and said that she had asked him how he could get through the two locked doors in the house. He looked at her but did not answer. She told him that the people on the other side would notice that he was missing. As soon as she told him that, he moved backward, out through the locked door, and just disappeared. She explained it as not really being he but his spirit.

During the years that I was in my religious organization, I had very little contact with my father's family. This was not due to their choice; I separated myself from them because I was passing religious judgment on them at that time. So we had almost no religious or spiritual conversations prior to this time.

After Heather died, I was so into my grief and struggle that I still had little contact with them. They had only known that I had left my religious organization just a year or so before. They were never sure why I left; they were just happy that they could have contact with me again. So, although we were family, we had not shared the same religious viewpoints. We had actually held contradictory positions for many years. Therefore, I was very pleased to have them relate these accounts to me.

I found it interesting that the people involved in their accounts usually moved backward and away from them. It reminded me of my mother's account with my father and of my own account with the faces of my father and Heather. So far, I have not come across any literature where others have specifically mentioned a backward moving away.

I learned a valuable lesson by opening up to my aunts. I had assumed that they would react differently than they did because of my mind set. God was again reminding me of the importance of not judging.

Although this is the last experience that I have chosen to include in this chapter, it is not the end of the experiences that people have shared with me. I have included the experiences that I think are relevant to my spiritual growth and that pertain to my family and to Heather.

As I approach the fifth anniversary of Heather's death, I have become more aware of how closely connected we all are and how closely we are interwoven with the oneness of the universe. I have come to realize that I am not as unique in this regard as I once secretly thought I was.

I am, however, unique in the manner of my discovery. I know that the experiences that I have encountered have helped me in my healing. I, therefore, hope that newly bereaved people can be comforted by my story.

I also hope that my journey gives courage to people who are in highly structured religious systems and feel the need to get out and move on. It does take courage, but the freedom is well worth it.

15

In Memory of Martti

*"Did I not tell you that if you would believe you would see
the glory of God?"* John 11:40

THIS BOOK HAD been in progress for several years.
When I started it, I didn't realize that we would lose another
loved one before it was published. This chapter is dedicated
to my husband's brother, Martti.

May 18, 1994, found me a little melancholy. We were going to have dinner at Kim's house that night. When we arrived, Kim said, "Mom, you seem quiet. What's the matter?"

I told her that I really wasn't sure why I was feeling so sad,
but it was Heather's prom anniversary date and perhaps I
was subconsciously remembering and reflecting on this.
May 18 had held tremendous significance twice already for

us. A third significant event was about to happen.

We had been at Kim's house for about an hour when we received a phone call. Martti had died just half an hour before. We did know this day was coming for him; we just didn't know that it would be that particular day.

I remembered when I had read my *Daily Word* that morning the text was, "In thy presence is fullness of joy." (Ps. 16:11) I had been thinking of Heather at that time. I had remembered it was her prom anniversary, and I had remembered the "calla-lily incident" from three years before. I reflected on her being in God's presence and on the word *joy* again. I never dreamed at that minute that by the end of this day I would be reflecting on Martti being in God's presence and filled with joy.

In November of 1993, we found out that Martti had metastasized cancer and would probably die within the year. He tried intensive radiation treatments in the attempt to save his life, but the cancer was too far advanced. Knowing that his death was getting near, we all spent more time with him. His checkups seemed to indicate that he was holding stable, and we were all hoping that we would have him through the summer months at least.

Martti loved the warm weather, and he loved cars and car shows. Walt planned on taking him to all the car shows in the area as soon as the weather broke and the shows began. Sadly Martti was able to see only one show; it, however, became part of an unusual set of coincidences.

The car show took place on the last weekend in April. Walt, Charlie, Joe, and some of the other guys in town took Martti to the show. He had a wonderful time. After the show, Charlie brought Martti over to his garage to show him the cars that he had been working on and the ones that were already finished. To quote Walt's words, "Martti was in his glory seeing all those old cars!"

Walt returned home very sad that night. Martti had taken off his favorite gold chain with the firebird emblem on it and had given it to Walt, telling him that he wanted him to have it. Walt was very emotional about this and was reluctant to take it. Martti insisted, and Walt arrived home that night with Martti's prized possession.

As Walt and I talked about this, we couldn't help but reflect on the connection this had with Heather. One of our automobiles is a Firebird—thanks to Heather. Let me explain.

One Saturday when I was finishing my M.S. in counseling, I was involved in an all-day workshop at the University (coincidentally, my professor was Gene). Walt and Heather decided that they didn't like my car and that I really needed a new one. They decided to just go and look to see what might interest me.

They both got carried away, however, and instead of just looking, Heather convinced Walt that I would love this new black Firebird, which she called "Kit." (Actually, I think Heather had plans for that car in the future!) They were able to complete all the necessary paperwork in that one day and drive home with the Firebird.

As a surprise, they took my old car from its parking space and replaced it with the Firebird. To make it even more special, they adorned the windshield with a dozen red roses.

Heather was to stay inside the car to watch my face, as well as to show me how to find the new switches. She thought the whole thing was hilarious; I almost had a nervous breakdown!

Imagine walking outside in the dark (after an intense all-day workshop) and trying to figure out why your car is not parked in the space that you left it in. At first, I thought that my car had been stolen and walked back inside to call the police. Someone suggested that I check again to be sure that I hadn't mistaken the parking spot.

I knew I had not, but I walked back outside to check anyway. I noticed that the car that was parked in my space had put its lights on and that this car also had my license plates on it. I really thought that I had lost it then. Heather roared with laughter. I didn't recover for days. The firebird and the roses would become much more significant in the years to come.

Martti loved our Firebird. He found the same emblem that is on our car hood and put it on his favorite gold chain. Walt never dreamed that years later he would wear that chain in memory of his brother.

As we reminisced over these events, we thought of the link that Heather and Martti had. The love of the Firebird was one link; so was the link of the disease, cancer. Another link would soon come.

Martti had lamented the death of his young niece. Heather's obituary notice was still on his desk—yellowed from time, but still there.

My niece, Kathy, called me about a week after the car show to tell me that she had had a dream of Heather the night before. She told me that Heather had appeared to her dressed all in black and that she was with Martti's uncle, Helge. She told me that neither of them said anything; they just stood there looking serious.

She asked me in what month Uncle Helge had died. I told her August. She then asked me if there were any significant dates in May for Martti, Helge, or Heather. I told her that other than Heather's prom date (May 18), no date in May was significant for any of them.

She then asked me if I thought that perhaps Martti would die in May and find Heather and Helge there to help him make the transition. I told her that I really didn't think so because I had just taken him for a checkup, and he was doing really well. I also told her that he was only taking two mild pain pills per day and that I assumed that the dosage would increase as his time drew nearer.

Since we couldn't think of what this dream could mean, we just recorded it and put it on hold. We shared this with other family members, but we did not tell Martti about the dream. (Sadly, on the night of May 18, we would all recall this dream.)

The same day that Kathy told me about her dream, Walt had stopped over to visit Charlie. He had not seen Charlie since the night of the car show when he and Martti had been in the garage. When he came home that day, he had an interesting story to tell me about Charlie.

After everyone had left the garage on the night of the car show, Charlie and Joe stayed for a while talking and cleaning up the garage. He told Walt that for some reason or another, the side door to the garage kept making a creaking noise.

He said that Joe began to tease Charlie and asked him if his garage were haunted. Charlie started laughing and kiddingly told Joe that he had a few female ghost friends. They both laughed at the whole idea. These two young "grease monkeys" weren't really believers in anything considered paranormal. That was about to change.

Charlie told Walt that shortly after he had said that to Joe, the song "The Rose" came on the radio. Charlie said to Walt, "I remember feeling really odd when that song came on the radio so soon after I had made that remark to Joe."

Charlie knew how much I loved that song. He also knew how special the charcoal rose sketch was to Walt and me. He loved Heather like a little sister and would let Heather come to his garage and borrow his classic cars. So, he immediately couldn't help but think of Heather.

Joe asked Charlie why he seemed serious and quiet, so Charlie started telling Joe about the connection between Heather and the rose. He told Walt that, as he was having this conversation with Joe, a piece of paper seemed to drift off one of the shelves. He and Joe walked over to see what the paper was. It was Heather's obituary notice (with her picture on it), now yellowed from being almost four years old.

Charlie told Walt that he could feel the hair on his arms

stand up. Joe became uncomfortable, and they decided to leave the garage. Both of them considered this a really weird coincidence.

Charlie gave the notice to Walt to show me, and he told Walt to tell me what had happened. It made such an impression in Charlie's mind that a week later when he came over to visit, he repeated the story to me. I could see by the expression on his face that he was truly impressed by what had taken place in his garage that night.

As Charlie explained, he didn't remember ever seeing the clipping in his garage. He said that Karen had probably cut the notice out when it originally appeared in the newspaper, but that she would have kept it in the house and not left it on one of the shelves in the garage. He further explained that he not only had no idea how the clipping got there, but, because he is so meticulous about keeping dust down in his garage, he cleans his shelves weekly (especially before painting a car). Therefore, he would have noticed the clipping before this time, he thought. He was truly stunned.

It was also an interesting coincidence that Charlie was with Walt and me when we got the phone call about Martti's death and that this would happen on the night of Heather's prom anniversary. Was Kathy's dream a sign that Martti would pass over on Heather's prom anniversary date?

Was the sign given to Charlie and Joe of the rose and the clipping further verification that Heather was a symbol for this coming event? Also, was Uncle Helge with Heather to indicate that they would be there for Martti to help him make the transition? Although it can't be proven, we all believe that Martti is with Heather and that she was there for him as he crossed over.

I recalled a conversation with Martti shortly before he died. He told me that although he was not a churchgoer, he definitely believed in some higher power. He told me that he wasn't sure how it worked, but that he knew that there was a higher dimension. I don't know how he knew this or why he believed this. Since it was a delicate subject at the time, I agreed with him and just added, "And when people get into that dimension, I've read that they go to the light." He just smiled at me.

The morning after Martti died, I woke up early to do my hour-long walk. I kept thinking of Martti and Heather and praying that they were together and in their glory. Suddenly I noticed a penny on the road. As I picked it up, I remembered Kevin's words from Heather, "A penny from heaven," and Kathy's words, "In God We Trust." Tears welled up in my eyes at this bittersweet reminder.

I whispered, "Hey, guys, be OK; I love you." As I walked back down my street, I saw Walt standing in the glass door. He turned up the radio quite loud. I listened closely and realized that I could hear the words from "Don't Know Much" playing. I was overwhelmed with the truth of the words. Love is all we really need to know. Any other information we acquire along the way is just frosting on the cake, teaching us how to apply this principle in our lives.

As I approached Walt, I saw that he was crying. I held up the penny. He smiled through his tears. He said that about half an hour before, Heather's other song, "When I'm Back on My Feet Again," had played. I told him that was about the time I had found the penny. We both smiled through our tears.

The road I walk on is well traveled and a penny along the way is likely, true. Yet I can honestly say that, in almost five years of walking that route, I don't recall ever seeing one and I never came home with one before. Also, why not a nickel, a dime, or a quarter; and why was it today?

Later that night, Elwood, Cynthia, and Marilyn stopped over to see us. Marilyn told me that she had also found a penny near her car that day. Cynthia noticed the firebird emblem on Walt's neck and remarked about it. Walt proceeded to tell her the story behind it. She then added another piece of interesting information about this symbol.

She told us that the firebird symbol also stands for the phoenix. She explained that the phoenix was a bird in Egyptian mythology that consumed itself by fire and then rose again renewed from its ashes. I had been unaware of this meaning and told her that I found this really interesting since Martti had decided to be cremated. She was surprised.

Did Heather and Martti subconsciously feel drawn to that symbol for a reason? We may never know, but one definition of the phoenix is a person or thing of unsurpassed beauty. The spirits of these two beloved ones truly fit this description. I pray that they can now soar like firebirds with this new freedom in spirit.

The following day I found another penny on my walk. This prompted a thought to cross my mind that became so strong I felt I had to act on it.

I remembered some three years before that my cousin Celia had urged me to say a prayer to St. Theresa of the Roses. I could not remember the words to the prayer or the protocol to follow, but from the depths of my being I begged God to forgive the "doubting Thomas" in me and to please give me a sign that Heather was with Martti and that they were both at peace.

I further asked to either hear the song "The Rose" or at least receive some form of a rose as an answer to this prayer.

As I returned from my walk, I picked up my mail before I entered the house. Two envelopes had roses on the return address labels and one card (from Elwood and Cynthia) had a vase of roses on it.

One of the envelopes was from my Aunt Gladys (Celia's mother) and contained a booklet entitled "A Pocketful of Miracles." The inside cover indicated that the twenty miracles cited were to show the power and compassion of our Lord. I was very moved by this gift and this answer.

When I called Cynthia to tell her what had happened, she added a bit more. She told me that she had especially looked for a card with a calla lily on it because of the connection to

Heather. She told me that she was really disappointed because she could not find one. Then she remembered how much the rose meant to us, so she decided to settle for the rose card. She didn't realize then that she would be part of the answer to my prayer.

Coincidence? Miraculous? Am I reading too much into events? *Webster's Dictionary* defines *miracle* as "an event that appears unexplainable by the laws of nature." Just because we can't explain something, doesn't mean that it does not exist. While it is true that those cards were already in my mailbox when I thought of saying this prayer, I had no way of knowing that the minute the thought passed through my head. The real question is what made that thought go through my head. I had only said that prayer once in my whole life, and that was over three years before.

What would motivate me to think that and then act on the thought? Perhaps God, knowing those rose symbols were already in my mailbox (and knowing my sadness), prompted the thought to pass through my head as a way of focusing me and then comforting me.

I'm reminded of a passage in Scripture that says, "Your faith has made you well; go in peace and be healed of your disease." (Mark 5:34) Isn't faith a belief?

Further, if the Bible (and modern medicine/psychology) points out that faith (belief) can physically heal a disease, why do we have such difficulty believing that our thoughts have real power? How many people are actively practicing a Bible-based religion, yet do not actually believe the power of this Bible passage?

I can't answer that for anyone but myself. But I know that belief can not only make you well; I know from experience that belief can also make you very ill. Many doctors believe this, too.

I thought of the *Daily Word* Scripture on the day that we held Martti's cremation service. It was, "Love Never Ends." (I Cor. 13:8) Is that so different from Heather's song, "Don't

Know Much," emphasizing that love was all there really was to know?

I reflected back to the day Heather died. The Scripture of the day in my former religion's *Daily Text* (which has an entirely different focus than the *Daily Word*) read, "Whether we live or we die, we belong to God." (Romans 14:8) Coincidence?

I didn't read that text until early evening on that day. I remember thinking how odd it was to have that Scripture being used for the day that she would die. I really didn't understand how this Scripture could be applied, since I had been taught and believed that Heather no longer existed, anywhere. Today, I am tremendously comforted by this. I know that she is with God—in another dimension.

A few days after Martti's death, Walt was in the local convenience store buying milk. He said that he was going through the change in his hand and dropped a quarter. When he bent down to pick up the quarter, he saw a penny beside it.

Had he not dropped the quarter, he would not have noticed the penny. To drive home the point, our newspaper carrier was standing in line and handed Walt an envelope. When he opened it later, there was a card with a beautiful calla lily on it.

As Walt related this to me, he said that he was not thinking of Heather or Martti while he was standing in line. It was not until he saw the penny that he instantly became focused on Heather and Martti. He said that as he stood there thinking about the two of them Phyllis (our newspaper carrier) handed him the envelope. As she explained to Walt, she was going to put the card in with our newspaper and had the card in her purse. Since she saw Walt in line ahead of her, she decided to hand it to him instead.

The timing was quite coincidental to Walt, however.

We really don't know Phyllis personally, so she would not have known of our special attachment to the calla lily. For

Walt, it was a very nostalgic moment to get the penny and the calla-lily card simultaneously. He said that it made him feel that Martti and Heather were there with him.

My mother-in-law (who is not interested in the paranormal) confided something interesting to me. She told me that she and my father-in-law (Martti's parents) were supposed to have gone camping at the time of Martti's death. She said that she kept feeling that she could not go. She didn't have any logical reason to feel that way, but she just refused to go. My father-in-law could not understand why and became annoyed with her.

Still, she refused to go. She said that she almost became physically ill just thinking of going. She could not understand why she felt the way she did. She just knew that she couldn't go and that was it. They canceled their plans. As a result, they were home when Martti called them just minutes before he died at his home on May 18, 1994.

As she told me this, I thought back to a few days after Heather died. My mother-in-law called our house and said that she could hear Heather's voice say, "Hello," just before our answering machine would pick up. Since Heather had never made any of our answering machine message tapes, it seems virtually impossible for her voice to be on the tape.

She insisted that she heard this on many occasions during the first year after Heather died. At the time, I was still involved in my religious structure and didn't give it much thought. If anything, I thought that she must be imagining it. I suddenly remembered this as she told me about feeling the necessity to stay home the day that Martti died.

Perhaps my mother-in-law (without her trying or knowing) was coming in contact with another dimension—one that none of us was aware of at that time. Perhaps, it is the fourth dimension that people refer to today.

16

Unfinished Business

"I tell you the truth," Jesus replied. "Before Abraham was born, 'I AM.' "   *John 8:58*

"I say to you that Elijah has already come but they did not recognize him"... the disciples perceived that he spoke to them about John the Baptist.   *Matthew 17:12-13*

I HAD NEVER believed in the theory of reincarnation. As a matter of fact, I considered the concept almost anti-God (surely at least anti-Christian). I just could not imagine going from a human to being born again as an animal.

It wasn't until I read the *Edgar Cayce Story of Karma* (Mary Ann Woodward), *Many Lives, Many Masters* (Dr. Brian Weiss), and *Many Mansions* (Dr. Gina Cerminara) that I began to take this theory seriously. I also came to realize that reincarnation and transmigration (humans to animals) were two very separate theories.

These books encouraged me to further research religion

and the Bible. I was still rather skeptical of this new theory, so I was pleasantly surprised to discover that the Bible (as well as many of the major religions of the world) did, indeed, encompass this theory. This new information was soon to become another important part of my spiritual picture. This theory also became a therapeutic aid in helping me to try to come to terms with the most difficult part of Heather's death.

I felt relieved when I read that the Cayce material had pointed out that it didn't really matter if an individual believed or doubted the theory of rebirth. This had nothing to do with a "salvation-type concept" based on the need to accept the doctrine. Instead, this could be a helpful concept in one's soul growth.

Cayce urged people not to dwell on the past or to brag about the past (if one had been important). The past could (if discerned) help us to see where we are going and to make wise choices in the future. In other words, we could grow from our past (if we were aware of it) regardless of when this past occurred. It could help us to discern what is important and to help us to choose (and we do choose) the most constructive way to respond in a given situation.

Coincidentally, I came across the book *Many Lives, Many Masters* through Gene, while I was still in bereavement counseling. He had no idea how reading this book would weave into my internal search for God. At that time, he was merely attempting to show me that people from all walks of life believed differently and that this was OK. But the book proved to be further verification that something greater than I could understand was working in my life. Again, Gene would be used as the catalyst for growth.

Since I deeply respected and trusted Gene (and he has an impeccable professional reputation), it seemed OK to take this book from him and read it. I had just finished it and had begun to give it some thought when the catalogue advertising the Cayce book on karma was accidentally placed in my mailbox. This is probably another reason why I ordered the book on karma along with the other books that I ordered on that day.

Because this theory was so controversial to my belief system, I'm not sure that I would have even considered it at this time in my life. It was the manner in which this theory was introduced (and reinforced) that led me to research the concept more thoroughly. The time spent in this research and the new information I acquired suddenly seemed to make the theory very acceptable in my life.

Although I started writing about Heather shortly after she died, I had no idea where the story would eventually take me. Nor did I always understand what was happening to me along the way. I just seemed to write (or tape record) bits and pieces of my time with her; at first, I could only see them as unrelated events in our lives.

Many times, I would feel at a loss for words; my mental engine just seemed to stall out. I would then coast for a while until the urge to talk or write came again.

This is by far the most difficult chapter for me to write, to understand, and, most of all, for me to accept. The difficulty comes in this way.

When Heather was first diagnosed with cancer, I knew that she would beat the cancer. I just knew it. I told her first physician that I would be the one to tell her of her diagnosis, and I preferred to do it alone and at home. He agreed and granted me that right.

The day I told her, I was extremely calm and confident. That was the day she also asked me for the *first* and *only* time, "Am I going to die because of this?" Her eyes quickly filled with tears and she gazed into my eyes intently.

I remembered very calmly looking her straight in the eyes and telling her, "No, you are not!" I said this because I believed it to be true. I knew that she would beat the cancer.

She had started to cry at first, but I noticed she was now intently staring at me. I knew, as a counselor, that if I didn't believe this myself that she would pick up on it and see right through me. But, the truth of the matter was that I was positive that cancer would not be the cause of her death. Fortunately, she believed me and she never asked me this again—never. (Notice I said asked and not told.)

Throughout the first year of Heather's treatment program, I felt as though I were on my initial roller-coaster ride; each climb, each turn, each descent produced fear and uncertainty in me. This made the roller-coaster ride especially rough for me. But, at least, I reasoned that I was learning and I was riding. Heather was just the opposite. Once she embraced her illness, she rode with it at the same roller-coaster pace. She was an inspiration to all around her (especially me).

For the most part, she liked all her medical caregivers. Some she especially loved, and they had a wonderful relationship with her. Some she felt were a bit crabby; but, all in all, she made friends of them. That is, all except one.

After Heather was chemically burned on her wrist by a leaking IV, it became necessary for her wrist to be repaired. The open wound would now become a danger to her for infection (especially when her white count was low). The doctor assigned to repair the wrist was not well received by Heather. This was the only time that she had actually requested another doctor.

She voiced this opinion to many of her caregivers, including the surgeon who had already performed three major surgeries on her. She told us that she did not feel comfortable with this new doctor and asked her regular surgeon why he could not perform the repair work instead of this new doctor. The surgeon told her that he could do the work and that he would speak to the doctors on her team. The team, however, preferred to have a plastic surgeon do the work, and Heather was not at all pleased with this decision.

I personally did not see this decision to be a problem, and I could not relate to Heather's feeling this way or voicing so strong an opinion. I knew that she had developed a very close relationship with her surgeon, and I realized that this was a natural request for her at this time. Her surgeon was an excellent and experienced doctor, and she had bonded strongly with him. I was assuming that this was probably a good part of the problem. This was approximately sixty days before she died.

Bone scans were also performed at about this time, and we were all delighted to learn that she was now cancer free. The remaining treatments would be given only as a precautionary measure to deter the return of the cancer.

The wrist repair surgery took place in August. Almost immediately, the wrist seemed to begin to deteriorate. The next course of chemotherapy was withheld until the doctor in charge of her wrist was sure that it was healing properly and that Heather was not at risk of getting an infection. When her white count reached a safe level and her wrist was said to be healing properly, permission for the chemotherapy was given.

Although the go-ahead was given in the second week of September, her wrist did not look as if it were healing properly and we voiced this opinion. We were informed that we were not medical people and that we were overreacting and that everything was fine. But, in reality, everything was not fine.

During Heather's last five-day IV chemotherapy treatment, nurses noted the wrist discoloration and oozing near the wound site and wrote this in their reports. When I brought her home on Saturday, a nurse friend changed the bandage and told me that I should get another opinion. She thought that the wrist was infected. I explained to her that Heather had just been seen by her doctor only a few hours before and that he said her wrist was fine and healing. He, therefore, released her to come home. My friend just shook her head.

On Monday, this nurse friend again looked at Heather's

wrist and told me that she was positive that the wrist was infected and to bring Heather back to the surgeon. I called the office and was given an appointment for the next day, Tuesday.

On Tuesday, the doctor assured me that her wrist was not infected and he refused to give me a prescription for an antibiotic. He told me to tell my nurse friend that she was not a specialist in this area and that she was only upsetting Heather and me.

Heather told him that she was experiencing greater discomfort and requested stronger pain medication. The doctor refused this request and cautioned us on the danger of taking unnecessary medication.

At this point, Heather became very upset with this doctor. He told her that she was overreacting and for me not to let her use her wrist. He told me that part of the problem seemed to be overuse of the wrist.

I explained to him (as he already knew) that her arm had been strapped in place in the hospital and that she had been mainly on bed rest since her release on Saturday. She had hardly used her wrist in over a week. Still, he said that she was fine and sent us home.

That night, Heather had a conversation with her cousin, Mike. He, in turn, related the conversation to his mother Pat. Pat was upset and called me. She said that we should really get another opinion as she, too, felt that the wrist was infected.

She knew of a highly respected specialist in this field, and she was able to get an appointment with him for Friday morning, September 21, at 11:00 a.m. Since Heather seemed so happy to get this appointment, I agreed that a second opinion would not hurt and that we would go.

Thursday I was up all night with Heather because her wrist was causing her tremendous pain. As soon as daybreak arrived, I called her doctor at 7:00 a.m. and demanded he see her.

The earliest appointment I could get was for that afternoon (Friday) at 1:30 p.m. I called my cousin Pat and suggested that we cancel her specialist until next week as Heather had been awake all night and I wanted her to try to get some rest before her doctor's appointment.

Heather came into the room and became very upset and insisted that we see Pat's specialist also. Pat agreed and urged me to keep this appointment. Since I could see how much this meant to Heather and since the appointments were two-and-a-half hours apart, it seemed reasonable that we could keep both appointments for this same day.

Pat's specialist was horrified. He photographed Heather's wrist and wanted us to give him feedback as soon as we could after seeing Heather's surgeon. Since this specialist was on his way out of town, he told us that he probably would not be able to see Heather again until Monday. He also told us that he was sure that Heather's doctor would admit Heather and put her on an intensive IV broad-spectrum antibiotic treatment.

At this point, I began having a sense of being in a bad dream and trying to wake up, but I seemed to be waking up a bit too slowly. By the time Heather's doctor saw her, it was 2:00 p.m. He was very cool to us. Pat, Heather, and I entered the examining room. I wanted Pat with me because I felt very nervous and wanted to be sure that I understood him correctly.

He still insisted that Heather was not infected. I then asked him to please call the oncology team to get her white count as I was sure that by now it would be close to zero. Hence, she would have almost no ability to fight an infection on her own. I wanted him to confer with them.

He refused and became very irritated with me. He told me that the call was unnecessary and that he would give Heather something (meaning a prescription for an oral antibiotic) to take care of any possible infection.

We asked him what the two black spots were on the border of the open wound. He merely replied, "I don't know." Since he seemed very calm and showed no obvious concern, I wondered if perhaps I wasn't just overtired and maybe I was overreacting.

I quietly and sadly expressed to him that I was very worried. He seemed kind for a moment and reassured me not to be worrisome (as he called it). He told me that there was really no danger and for me to try to relax. As I said, he actually seemed to be kind at that moment.

Pat asked him to give Heather a shot because of the pain. Again, he seemed kind and told us that he did not keep anything like that in his office, but that he would give her a prescription for a narcotic to make Heather more comfortable. Finally, I thought, we were getting someplace. He examined her wrist slowly and put silverdene around the wound just in case there were any bacteria present (as he explained). He then bandaged the wrist back up, gave us some prescriptions, and told us to go home.

Once again, he told me that I was overreacting and that there was no reason for me to be "worrisome" over this. He was so sure she was OK that he told me he would not see Heather again until the following Wednesday.

Pat and I reluctantly and silently drove home. Heather just quietly slumped back on the seat and I knew that she was very tired. Although we felt that we were finally getting someplace, we still both felt very uneasy. We stopped to fill her prescriptions and to give Heather her first dose of medication in the car.

We finally returned back home. It was now after 5:00 p.m.

Mary and Erick were very close to Heather and came over to cheer her up and to have dinner with us. Heather felt too ill to eat, and Mary kept her company while I put the meal together.

Heather opted to lie down very early in the evening. Usually, she is a "night owl," but I reasoned that she was extra tired due to losing last night's sleep. By 8:15, the pain medication did not seem to be helping her so I gave her another dose (this was only three-and-one-fourth hours after the first dose instead of the four hours prescribed). I could see the pain very visible in her face.

By 10:00 p.m., Heather was requesting more pain medication. I knew that this was far too soon to give her another pain pill. She became very distraught over my refusal and began to sob. I held her close to me to try to comfort her, and I immediately noticed that she was hot.

I panicked! I knew a rise in temperature was a very dangerous sign. I suddenly realized that the doctor had not even bothered to take her temperature that afternoon. I quickly ran to take it. The thermometer read 102°.

I knew only too well that this was a very bad sign for an infection. To hell with the surgeon! I paged the oncology doctor on call. When he finally got back to me, he immediately asked, "What's her temperature?"

When I told him that it was 102°, he said, "You need to bring her in immediately!" I told him that I had just been to see the surgeon hours ago and I explained to him what had transpired in the office visit.

Silence came on the line. When he spoke again, he told me to bring Heather in immediately and to bring her into the emergency unit instead of her regular unit. My heart sank; I knew that we had almost an hour's drive to get there. I seemed to sense that time was a big factor here.

We all piled into the car, and Erick drove as quickly as he could to the hospital. I could hear him cursing under his breath. I knew that he, too, was frightened for Heather.

As we entered the emergency room, people seemed to gather around us. They had been told to expect us. The doctor on call examined Heather's wrist and said, "This looks like dead meat; we need to get a culture." Mary's face went white. I knew how much Erick and Mary loved Heather also. An atmosphere of concern seemed to envelop the room.

The doctor took Heather's temperature—almost 104°!

My heart began pounding so hard with fear that it was difficult for me to keep my composure for Heather. The doctor on call ordered her to be immediately put on a broad-spectrum IV antibiotic. He then had her sent up to her regular floor.

I have constantly been plagued by this particular twenty-four-hour scenario. Why were two doctors concerned about a culture, yet the other one was not? Why were two doctors concerned about the rise in temperature, yet the other one was not? Why were two doctors concerned about a zero white count, yet, the other one was not?

I can't begin to even count the number of times these questions have raced through my head. Why? How could the obvious be so unobvious to a doctor who successfully practices in two large hospitals? As of today, I still do not have an answer that satisfies me. Perhaps there is none to be found.

Because another specialist had examined Heather and was concerned about her progress, an investigation did take place. Medical errors were discovered and disciplinary action was taken. Some may call this justice. I still cannot.

I have often thought about the set of circumstances that happened in that twenty-four-hour period. Suppose I had canceled Heather's other appointment on that fatal Friday? If I had done that, no photographs would have been taken and no other testimony could have been given—at least none of such a credible nature.

Consider, also, that within hours after that office visit, Heather would never be able to walk out of that hospital again. She would never have been able to voice her dissatisfaction to another expert, and he would never have been able to examine her. Only hours separated these events. Why? Is this just an uncanny set of bad circumstances? Or is it just possible that this has roots and meaning in another dimension? Perhaps, even in another lifetime?

Of course, I do not have a concrete answer for all these

questions. I, personally feel that it has a much deeper meaning than I can, as yet, discern.

Consider, too, that Heather made it through the biopsy surgery; she made it through chemotherapy; she made it through her first rib removal; she made it through more chemotherapy; she made it through the infected porto-cath removal; she made it through more chemotherapy; she made it through an emergency appendectomy during her wrist repair; she made it through more chemotherapy; she came out cancer free on her last bone scan (which her autopsy verified).

Why, in God's name, did she have to die to a lousy and obvious infection while being treated by a reputable doctor?

Why? Why would she have to go through all that suffering only to die of something so obvious? And why did she immediately react so negatively to this particular doctor?

I believe that I will probably go to my grave without an answer. The whys still plague me. I have so wanted to put closure to this aspect and yet I really cannot. Since Heather put this in motion, I feel that it is "unfinished business" for her. Or, perhaps, it is even for me.

One night while I was really in a dilemma over this, I had a vivid dream of Heather. In the dream, I was trying to find her in a place that resembled a hospital/school type of facility. Walt and I had to sneak into the main office to look at the records to find out the number of the room she was in. We seemed to be dropping a lot of 3" x 5" cards from a small file on a nurse's desk. Finally, we found her card. (For the sake of confidentiality, I will change the numbers and the name here.)

We finally found out that she was located in room 628.

We quickly got into the elevator and pushed the button. The elevator doors opened up, but instead of being on the sixth floor, we seemed to be on the eighth.

We stayed in the elevator and pushed the button again.

The elevator did not move, but the other side of the elevator seemed to open up. This time we saw the number six and knew that we were on the sixth floor.

We began to run down the corridor, past medical personnel. Suddenly, the numbers stopped at 620. We panicked! There was no 628. I began to sob.

Then, we noticed that if we crossed the corridor, the numbers began again at 622 and went up to 628. We ran across the corridor and ran to her room. We pushed open the door, but it seemed to open into a huge auditorium and it was filled to capacity with people. Every seat was taken and the auditorium floor was filled with people moving about. We were overwhelmed.

We began to descend slowly, row by row, downward toward the auditoriums' ground-level floor. We searched each row carefully looking in every seat for Heather, but there was no Heather to be found.

Down, down, slowly down, we anxiously searched for her.

We finally landed on the ground level and stood in the middle of a crowd of people all walking around. We looked at each of them. Still I could not find Heather. I started to cry.

Suddenly, to the right of us, we noticed another section of the room. We walked toward this area and realized that it was almost a duplicate of the section we had just left. We were now on the bottom level, and we could see rows and rows of auditorium seats going up, up, up, almost out of sight. Still we could not see Heather.

We began to ascend slowly. Row by row, we would check, seat by seat, to see if we could see her. But there was still no Heather. I could feel myself being weighted down with despair. It seemed like hours went by as we ascended row by row and checked seat by seat of this fully packed section.

Finally, we seemed to be approximately three rows from the top. I stopped to catch my breath and to scan the last few rows. Suddenly something grabbed and squeezed my heart. There, on the aisle seat of that last row, sat my beautiful child, Heather. My heart quickened!

As I gazed at her, she looked the way she had on the day that she had first cut her real hair short because she was losing so much from the chemotherapy. I just kept staring at her and praying that this moment would never end and that I would enter into eternity with this feeling. Words can never adequately express my emotion at this moment.

I gazed intently into those beautiful blue eyes. She was looking at me in the way that people would look at someone they had noticed in a crowd and realized that the person was too far away to catch their attention. But I also knew from this stare that she had watched us every step of the way as we ascended closer and closer to her.

As our eyes fully engaged, she gave me the sweetest and most innocent "childlike" smile that I had ever seen on her face. I softly whispered, "Heather, Heather, I can't believe that we have finally found you!" I began to sob.

I advanced quickly toward her and bent down to embrace her in my arms. I could almost smell her. Although she was life-sized and resembled the way that I remembered her looking, a strange thing began to happen.

As my arms advanced around her and my embrace tightened, she seemed to be getting smaller and more condensed to hold. I stopped for a minute and softly asked her, "Can you walk or do you want me to carry you?"

She seemed already a part of me and she whispered to me, "Carry me." I immediately tightened my grip on her so as not to chance losing her again. Yet, as I did this, she became smaller and smaller and more and more condensed. Suddenly she seemed to be absorbed right into me. I began to cry.

Immediately, I was awake and deeply sobbing. It was such a painful loss to wake up. Walt woke up to my sobbing and asked me what was wrong. I told him about my dream.

The next morning Cynthia called and I told her about the dream. We both cried. That morning I repeated the dream account to Pat, Marilyn, and Ginny. They, too, were moved.

It had been a while since I had a dream about Heather.

It left me extremely sad and nostalgic. I called Gene to talk to him and to tell him about my dream. He, too, shared my sadness.

Later that day, I went to see my mother and she told me what had happened to her a few nights before. She said that she had awakened to Heather sitting on the side of her bed; at first she thought that she was dreaming. But the loud sound of her own voice had made her fully conscious. She wondered why she was talking and sensed that she was conversing with someone.

She opened her eyes while she was talking and she suddenly stopped short. She told me that Heather was sitting beside her just staring at her. My mother could not seem to remember what the conversation was about. She just felt strongly that Heather had been trying to tell her something.

Suddenly Heather reached out to take my mother's hand. My mother extended it for a minute and then said, "My God, Heather, it's you!" She then pulled her hand back quickly. With that, Heather seemed to exit back away from her and out the wall.

Since my mother had been ill lately, I asked her if she thought that Heather may have come to see if she were ready to go to the other side. My mother thought for a second, then told me that it could be that because she was feeling tired, she probably would have accepted the offer.

I told her that if she had really wanted to go she would probably have actually gone. I told her that perhaps her work on this side was not yet finished. She thought about this for a minute and said, "I think you are right." Although we aren't sure what her unfinished work is, nonetheless, she is still here and doing quite well.

When I came home from my mother's house that day, I

picked up my mail. There was a letter from the specialist who had seen Heather on that last Friday. He wrote me that he had gone as far as he could possibly go on his own and that he had received further advice from an expert who would help us to resolve this matter. He asked me to call him right away. I called him and made an appointment to see him two days later.

I called Pat to ask her to go with me as I had only been there that one time and was not sure how to get there. She told me that she would be out of town that day and, since Cynthia knew the area quite well, she would give the directions to her.

Cynthia offered to drive since I felt nervous. I told her that I would recognize the building when we got there because it was very distinctive looking. We chatted about the dream and what the possible implications could be. We finally came to the crossroads where the specialist's office was located. As we looked at the large white house, in big gold numbers and letters was the partial address: 620 Heaven (it was Heaven's Way).

Both Cynthia and I gasped at the huge gold sight in front of us. Was my dream telling me that this specialist at 620 was as far as he could go and that we would have to go farther (across town, actually) to complete the heavenly course? Was Heather telling me to carry her farther because something needed to come out?

Why would I have had that dream on the night before I would get the letter? Why would the numbers be so symbolic? Several people knew about my dream before the letter arrived.

The letter was dated the day before (which was the night of my dream), and it arrived one day later at the normal time in my mailbox. I would have had no way of knowing this before I received my mail.

Yet the combination of that dream and the coincidental arrival of that letter made me know for certain that it was now essential for me to carry to completion the unfinished business which Heather had started. My dilemma was now resolved. I would carry out her last earthly wish.

I have always said, "Heather's task," but the more I read and learn, the more I realize that there is also some meaning in this for me or I would not be involved in this task. Is this some kind of karmic lesson I'm involved in?

As of today, I still do not have a positive answer to this. But I don't believe that it was only a coincidence that found Heather setting something in motion on the last day she could function outside of a hospital.

It has always been difficult for me to accept things when I cannot understand them. Therefore, it is natural for me to search for meanings and for answers. Yet I wonder if I will ever know the meaning of this whole thing. Is it for me to know?

I have finally come to believe that if it is meant for me to know, I will get the answer. I have grown to believe and accept that a power far greater than we can comprehend does exist. It is through the accepting of this fact that I have become tremendously healed.

17

Resurrection

"Awake, O Sleeper, and arise from the dead." Ephesians 5:14

WHEN HEATHER DIED in the flesh, I died with her; my body seemed to remain here, but the person I once was had ceased to exist. I felt dead; I wished I were dead; and I could not imagine ever feeling any different.

I would never have believed then that years later I would emerge into the person I am today, writing a book with this viewpoint. It would have been virtually impossible for me to do this. Yet, I have changed.

Time is an essential element. Grieving is a process, not an event. Unfortunately grieving requires time. To anyone who may be in the earliest stages of grief, my heart aches for you. I pray that you realize that time can definitely heal you. I know because I've been there.

I also urge you to do what is sometimes referred to as "grief work." Yes, sad to say, even grieving has work involved. I believe this work is essential in healing.

As I look back to the year 1990, I can still recall the horror. Yet I can now recognize the path that was evolving for me. I have come to know that there is something greater than I can see or understand, and I have come to accept that.

In July of 1990 our state offered a retirement package that I qualified for. Although I had earned enough years of service to retire, I had no intention of doing so at that point in my life. I had been urged by friends, however, to make an appointment with the retirement board just to see what the package included. The appointment was scheduled for the last week in July.

Since the counselors in the vocational school had already taken the retirement package, I applied for and was granted a vocational counseling position. I was thrilled.

I had transferred from teaching to counseling two years previously and I loved my new position. However, I had always wanted to be a vocational counselor. Finally, I had realized my dream.

To make this position even more appealing, I would be working again with some of my close friends. Jimmy and I had worked together in the business department years before, and we were a great team together. He had now become the acting director of the vocational facility (and eventually would become the director). So I was doubly thrilled.

Since Heather's treatments (at that time) were to be finished around the end of September, I reasoned that this would be a good time for me to start a new position. Perhaps this would give me a new focus in life. I decided to accept the position and to cancel my retirement appointment.

It's a good thing that I mentioned this to Ginny, as well as to Elwood, before I canceled my appointment. Ginny urged me to keep the appointment. Elwood also insisted that I keep it and that I consider all the options available to me at that time. I was reluctant to do this, but I decided to go in and at least talk to the retirement counselor. I found out that this counselor had lost a child to cancer and that she had had the same doctor and hospital that Heather did.

When she realized what I was contemplating, she urged me to take the package. She told me that even if Heather were in remission that it was still possible for her to relapse. She told me that if I really wanted to go back into teaching/counseling after Heather was finished with her treatments, I could always work in a private school. She strongly urged me to reconsider this carefully as there was now only one week left in which to decide.

When I came home later that day, I discussed this with Walt and Elwood. Ginny called that evening and urged me to take the package. I can honestly say that if it weren't for Elwood and Ginny, I might not have taken early retirement.

I thank God that I listened to them. In less than two months my life would become so dramatically altered that I would not have been able to emotionally function in my "dream job."

I was sad the day I went in to give my notice. I had loved the Chariho school system. I swear they employ the best people in the world. Also, I had so loved my students. I still have friendships with those whom I had in class some twenty years ago. It was really sad to say goodbye to such a wonderful part of my life. Yet I would come to learn that it really was time.

Time was the gift that I was being given. Without this time, I never would have been able to do the research and thinking that would become so crucial to my healing and survival. I obviously had no control over the state offering the retirement package at that time. I was also blessed by the fact that I qualified for the package and that friends of mine stepped in and urged me to take it. I would never have been able to give quality time and consideration to the young people who would have been assigned to me. Several years would pass before I even felt the desire to interact on this level again.

As the years passed, I could see the healing that was taking place within me. Time was easing the pain. Time was also allowing me to sift through and to integrate all of the new information that I had acquired.

The waves of horror, anger, and sadness were no longer sweeping over me with hurricane force, knocking me down. The storm was finally subsiding and the waves were coming and going with a gentler, more soothing pace. Yes, the waves still come—but I have finally learned to swim in the waves.

One of my favorite proverbs is, "If you give people a fish, you feed them for a day; but if you teach them to fish, they can feed themselves for a lifetime."

This adage was one that I had always applied to others. Now I could see the application for myself. I was finally learning to peacefully fish and to acquire knowledge that would help me in this particular lifetime. I didn't look to others any longer to supply me with my answers (my fish). I have decided to fish on my own.

Because of my particular religious background, people will sometimes ask me if I believe the world will still come to an end in this particular lifetime and if I am frightened by this (as I once was). My answer to this is twofold.

While I believe that we are living during crucial times, perhaps on the edge of a new enlightenment, I think that many people are overly focused on the approaching end of this millennium. We shouldn't get caught in the negative.

Although Cayce believed that Christ's second coming would occur in this century, he did not predict a physical and total end to this earth. He pointed out that the future is not fixed or predetermined and that our daily thoughts and deeds are continually shaping what's ahead.

He further urged people to consider how the second coming takes place, physically or in consciousness. The reader must evaluate this for himself or herself, individually.

I urge people to consider this issue carefully. There are many options available today, including hoarding food and ammunition underground, being "born again" or "saved" somehow, being picked up by a flying saucer, or perhaps joining a particular religious institution to insure your salvation (like I did).

In that way, you can let someone else do your thinking for you. Then you have a scapegoat in case that course does not turn out to your benefit. But what does it fester within you? Fear. Be careful; I've been there; don't let anyone decide for you.

Some of the most powerful words ever spoken by Jesus in regard to the second coming are seldom mentioned by groups who have all the answers. I urge you to keep these words before you.

Luke 21:27-28 says, "They will see the Son of Man coming with power and glory . . . raise yourselves erect and lift your heads up . . . your deliverance is near."

Whether this coming is a physical event, a spiritual event, or a consciousness-raising event, and whether this comes as an individual shedding of your body or a cataclysmic shedding of many bodies at once, you are more than just your body.

Consider also whether one dies in a horrendous end-of-the-world scenario, or whether one dies of cancer or some other disease or disaster, one will still die alone. Just because one may be standing (or sitting) with hundreds of people all dying together does not make one's own personal death experience either better or worse. We each still experience birth and death as a unique individual experience.

I think the more important issue here really is, do we survive physical death in some form? If so, what is the criterion for this salvation? I believe it is simply love.

I used to worship a God of judgment. I thought that He was mainly concerned with what formal religion a person believed was intellectually correct and I thought that if you didn't understand God correctly, you would be damned forever. I now realize that if that were the case, you would have to become almost smarter than God in order to explain Him correctly. If that were true, I am convinced that none of us would make it.

I no longer picture myself standing before the throne of this supreme God of Love and explaining to Him that I was striving hard to love my fellow humans (instead of intellectually explaining God) and have God condemn me to damnation for doing that. I can no longer view God like that.

I have changed tremendously since Heather's death. In essence, I once believed that my God wanted intellectualism; and I would have condemned you and passed judgment on you if you did not believe as I did. I would not have voiced this thought out loud in those days, and I would have been tactful in the way I worded something. But, in essence, that is the crux of my old belief system.

Before Heather died, I never would have believed that I would think like I do today. Yet I do, and I am a lot more peaceful in this belief. The gift of time has truly changed me.

I now take time daily to walk and to experience nature. To me, walking is very therapeutic. I also take time to focus daily on something spiritual and to meditate and pray. I use the *Daily Word* to help me focus as I start each new day.

My prayer and meditation routine is very informal. I tend to follow Cayce's simple meditation procedure of relaxing and focusing on love. Some people like a more structured routine. That's OK for them. I am just in a different place than they are, and that's OK, too.

Just before Martti was found to be terminal, I had decided to become a member of the local hospice team. I had seen an ad in the newspaper and had cut the ad out because I knew that Ginny was interested in becoming a hospice volunteer. I planned on showing her the ad. But, as the days went by and I kept looking at this ad, I felt a desire to do this for myself.

I signed up for the next workshop and began my training. I didn't realize then that my first patient would be Martti. The day after I completed the training, we learned that Martti was terminal; his radiation treatments were not enough, and the cancer was too far metastasized for further treatments.

I was the one who called the doctor to have him referred to hospice. As a result, Martti's last wish (to die at home) could be realized. Although I worked with Martti more as a family member than I did as a hospice volunteer, the training that I had received was very valuable to me in this endeavor. So was my own personal experience.

Since I had not been familiar with the hospice program before this time, I was unaware of what they believed. I had read *Final Gifts* by two hospice nurses, but thought that this was more about their personal experiences with people and their own individual beliefs. I received a pleasant surprise on my first day of training.

Each participant was given a folder with all the material that would be covered during our training sessions. As I looked through the folder, I came across a booklet entitled *When Death Is Near*. This booklet helps families to understand the physical changes that occur in the body when a person is near death. But to me, it also validated my new concept of spirituality and life after death.

Consider that this booklet is published by the VNS (Visiting Nurse Services) and is given out by the hospice team. In several places in this ten-page booklet, reference is made to the spirit releasing from the body. It also brought out that the dying may be found talking to unseen people or with those who have already died. This information is presented in such a manner that one would consider this everyday normal activity.

Imagine if I had signed up for this course five years previously! I would have quit. Yet, here was the medical profession validating experiences that some would consider to be crazy. However, to the group of professionals who work with the dying, it's quite normal and acceptable. I greatly appreciated receiving such information in this manner. It became further verification to me that I was, indeed, on the right path.

I have also come to appreciate the value of volunteering. Obviously, in my profession, I was paid to perform counseling services, and there is nothing wrong with this concept. But, for me, volunteering became a therapeutic part of my healing, just as walking, praying, and meditating have.

Everyone's path is different. Time has given me the ability to do this now, and I feel that it is God's direction. Jesus was right. There truly is more happiness in giving than there is in receiving.

This is true because they are actually interrelated. When you give from your heart simply because you want to give (and no wage or reward is intended), the gift of love that seems to come back to you is overwhelmingly wonderful. It's sort of like a boomerang effect.

Nothing or no one can give us or buy us this feeling. It comes from the heart, from inside of us, and it is a part of us. Yes, we were created in God's image and we were created to love and to create love. Nothing else really matters. That is where I am today.

True, the Geri that I once was died with Heather on that brutal day in September of 1990. It was years before the resurrection was to be complete. Today, a new person lives in that physical body. I do believe that when this physical body has served its purpose here on the earth, its spirit will separate and go into the spirit realm.

While I am here, however, I'm going to try to live just one day at a time. I'm trying to learn to seize each moment and to live in the here and now. I pray that I can remember each day to appreciate this gift of life and to try extra hard to love my fellow humans. To live my life with love is the gift that I can give back.

18

Boston, and Then Some

"Set your hearts on spiritual gifts, especially the gift of speaking God's message."   *I Corinthians 14:1*

E A R L Y I N T H E winter of 1994, I began to put this book into typed form using my journals and recorded messages. I did this to save my sanity since the New England coast was hit with seventeen major snow storms and I was often confined to the house. I viewed this as an opportunity to begin to put this book into order.

I had just finished the chapter in which I explained how I had come into contact with the readings of Edgar Cayce. A few days later, as I was working on the next chapter, my husband brought in the mail. That day it contained a yellow sheet of paper from the A.R.E. Press called "The Good

Word," vol. 3, number 1, Winter 1994.

I was suddenly jolted into awareness by a six-paragraph article entitled "Wanted: Your Book Proposal." I hadn't thought of seeking a publisher yet, since I only had a few chapters finished at this point. I wasn't even aware that A.R.E. actually published books. I knew that they sold books and had ordered from their catalogue, but I did not know that they actually published books until this yellow paper arrived.

I remember immediately thinking to myself, "I wonder if I am supposed to send a proposal in to them." I finished reading this paper and immediately sent for their author's guidelines.

I followed the instructions and mailed the first two chapters and an outline to the editors. I was very pleased when they expressed interest in the first two chapters and asked to see more. It's significant to note the date of the letter in which this request came. It was May 19, 1994, just one day after Martti had died. Since I had only approximately 100 pages completed and I was not emotionally able to write at that point, I sent A.R.E. what I had typed so far.

It was probably close to September when I finally finished the book and sent the rest of the material to Ken, an editor at A.R.E. Press. Now the book would either be accepted or rejected. (Obviously, this chapter was not yet included, as you will see.)

The weekend of September 30-October 2 found me in Boston with Cynthia, Marilyn, Celina, and Kim attending the Body and Soul Convention sponsored by *New Age Journal* and *Interface*. The conference was wonderful.

It was, however, larger than was originally expected (over 1,700 people from forty states and three foreign countries) and, therefore, some of the workshops were held outside of the hotel. I was irritated to learn that my first workshop (with Kim) on Saturday morning would be held at some large church.

Since I had seldom been to Boston and since I am intimidated by large cities, I considered changing my first session and going to a different workshop. I noticed, however, that Brian Weiss, whom I had been wanting to meet for several years now, was also scheduled to be at this same church later on that day. I would have to find this place eventually, so it might as well be now.

Fortunately, it was only down the street one block from the side entrance of our hotel and the weather was nice. Kim and I went to that first session, and we were glad we did. Matthew Fox, who also struggled with his religious structure, was a wonderful lecturer, and we gained a lot from this workshop.

As Kim and I left the church and walked down the stairs, Kim asked me if I knew where a certain hotel was. I hardly knew Boston, so I'm not sure why I turned my head to see the street sign. But, as I did, my heart froze for a second. I looked at the street sign. It was Newbury Street. Kim looked at my face and said, "Ma, what's the matter?"

Tears welled up in my eyes as I told her that the last time that I had been in Boston, I had been on Newbury Street with Heather buying her a wig from a shop called Avalon. Heather's death anniversary had just been a week ago, and I still had a calla lily in the house from this observance (as well as some on her grave).

Of all the places to be in this huge city, why would I be standing at the corner of Newbury Street. I remembered walking around this same corner, along this same street with Heather as we went to get some lunch with my cousin Pat.

Now, five years later, I had returned with my other daughter. This time it involved a search for spiritual reinforcement. I found this so sadly nostalgic.

Kim and I shared this with the others when we returned for the second session. The third session found Kim, Celina, and me returning to this church.

As we got closer to the steps of the church, we noticed a foreign vendor selling flowers on the church steps. What was he selling? Calla lilies!

Kim, Celina, and I were speechless. It was difficult for me to stay focused now even though I had so wanted to see Brian Weiss in person. Celina leaned over to me and whispered, "If the flower vendor is still there when we leave (in two hours), I'm going to buy you a calla lily for the hotel room."

Sure enough, he was still there. Kim also noticed that he was selling a combination bouquet of roses and calla lilies, and she bought one for her room in remembrance of her sister. As we returned to join Marilyn and Cynthia, they, too, were stunned by this remarkable coincidence.

We quickly went to our rooms to put the flowers in water. I couldn't help but think of the calla lily at home in memory of Heather as I sat in my hotel room looking at the one that Celina had purchased for me. I reflected on how unusual it was to find one. I had to order my flowers in advance because calla lilies are not in season that time of year. Yet this vendor had lots of them. Even more amazing was that the vendor was right at the corner of Newbury Street where Avalon was located. It's also interesting to note that we never did see another vendor selling flowers during the rest of that weekend, no matter where we walked in Boston.

Heather was heavy on my mind now. The next lecture Cynthia and I attended was given by Jean Shinoda Bolen. When she was introduced, they cited her book, *Crossing to Avalon*. Cynthia and I looked at each other. She whispered, "Maybe we are supposed to read that." I nodded.

The next morning, I seemed to be the only one in our group scheduled to hear Bernie Siegel. The room he was speaking in was packed to capacity, and the divider had to be removed in order to accommodate the rest of the people waiting to hear him. I scanned the room quickly to see if there were any vacant seats toward the front.

I was in luck. Approximately ten rows from the stage was one vacant seat and it was right on the aisle. Great! I hurried to the seat and asked the young woman next to it if it were being saved. She smiled and said, "No." I sat down.

As we sat waiting for Bernie Siegel to take the stage, this young woman and I began chatting. She asked me what workshops I had attended so far and became interested in the one on Brian Weiss. She told me that she had just begun her spiritual journey and was rather confused about the doctrine of reincarnation. She asked me if I could briefly explain what I thought the doctrine to be.

I explained it to her the way I had once explained it to Kim. One day while Kim was having difficulty trying to blend theories of past lives with the person who she is today, she asked me, "How would I know who I really am if I have been other people at different times? Which person would I really be?" She was actually quite upset over this dilemma.

I told her that we have always been the same unique souls (spirits) since our moment of creation by God in His image. We have, however, elected to play various roles at various times in history in order to achieve soul growth.

Sometimes we play the role of a man; sometimes we play the role of a woman. Sometimes we play the role of a white person; sometimes we play the role of another race or skin color. Sometimes we are rich; sometimes we are poor; and sometimes we are in between.

It's like a movie star who plays many roles or characters in the course of his/her career. Actors and actresses are not the characters that they are playing. They are always the same movie stars in this lifetime. Yet many of these professional actors have stated how they grow and learn from the roles that they play. They stress that it is often hard work to achieve the performance they desire to give. It's similar to that idea, only far more spiritual.

I told her to view her soul as taking on a body in order to interact with others while on this earth. This body is like a vehicle or a car. I drive the "Geri car" and Walt drives the "Walt car" and Kim drives the "Kim car" and so forth. But we are not the car. We only reside in the vehicle for a period of time in order to accomplish a purpose or reach a goal.

When that purpose has been accomplished, we will exit the car (in spirit); the vehicle will have served its purpose for this particular lifetime and, henceforth, will no longer be needed. The car has died (so to speak); we have not. We go back to the spirit world as the same spirit, but with more soul growth. It's similar to going to school. It is hoped that we are a bit smarter after a few more years of lessons.

I remembered that Kim could relate to this explanation so I asked this young woman if it made sense to her. She smiled and told me that it did. I then asked her about the workshops that she had attended.

She immediately talked about the one she had attended with Bernie Siegel the afternoon before. She told me that he had asked them to draw a symbol of what they felt represented them at this point in their lives. She then opened her notebook and showed me an 8-1/2" x 11" picture of a beautiful red rose. I gasped!

When she questioned my reaction, I told her about Heather and my connection with the rose. Tears filled her eyes, and she shared with me a very sad and personal account of why she felt the rose represented her at this point in her life. Tears filled both of our eyes as Bernie Siegel took the stage.

I had never met this woman before, yet our souls touched each other deeply that day as we shared personal and sensitive thoughts. Why had the one empty chair been near a young woman with long blonde hair and blue eyes—who would show me a rose? I knew the correctness of my path as I sat there.

The whole weekend was a wonderful time of affirmation for me (as well as the rest of our group). I was then approximately four years into my spiritual journey, a journey that began because of an apparition and a dream. I was also feeling much more secure about what I was learning.

All of us felt so connected after this conference—not only to each other but to the oneness of the universe. Seeing all these seekers at one conference and listening to all those great researchers really helped to reinforce the notion that something else was truly out there. And we weren't the only ones who knew this.

I came home with my calla lily and put it in a vase on my kitchen counter. The other calla lily to commemorate Heather's memorial was still alive and doing well on her bedroom bureau. I felt very strongly that my book would be published by A.R.E. Press. I tried to be patient and wait for the answer.

Approximately a month after this conference, I received a response from a letter I had written to a psychic in Ohio.

I had seen Patricia Mischell on the Jerry Springer talk show and was so impressed that I wrote to her.

Since it had been some time ago, I had actually forgotten about this until her letter arrived. She explained that there had been an overwhelming response to her appearance on this show and thousands of people had written to her. Many of them (like myself) had forgotten to include a self-addressed, stamped envelope. Hence, the long delay. The letter indicated that it was possible to get a telephone reading from her, so I decided to have one.

My appointment was for Wednesday, December 14, 1994. I was so excited that I could hardly wait until this day arrived. I no longer doubted that there were gifted people who could communicate with another dimension. I was curious as to what she would be able to tell me.

The day before my reading, Walt came home with a strange look on his face. He told me that he had just had a weird experience in his new car. He had been driving home from the dentist when he noticed a ball of light moving within the car.

At first he thought that either his watch or his ring was picking up the sun's reflection and moving the reflection throughout the car. He kept trying to determine how this could be because the ball of light seemed to be moving independently in the car. He quickly became aware that this phenomenon was not being caused by the watch, the ring, or any other reflection. It was just a ball of light moving about.

He pulled off the road into a shady spot to see what could possibly be causing this phenomenon. The ball of light (about the size of a quarter) just kept independently moving about. Suddenly it just moved right past him and out the window. He was stunned!

When he told me about this, I asked him what his first thought was when he realized that the ball of light moved on its own. Tears came into his eyes as he quietly murmured, "Heather." I had suspected that Walt was really falling in love with this new car since he was hardly driving the Firebird any more. So, I asked him if he were feeling guilty about having a new car—as if he were deserting Heather. As he nodded in agreement, Heather's song ("When I'm Back on My Feet Again") started to play on the radio.

We both started to cry. I tried to comfort Walt by telling him that maybe Heather was reassuring him that it was OK for him to go on with his life and enjoy new things since material items were no longer of interest to her in the realm that she was in. He agreed. Nonetheless, we were sort of baffled by the ball of light.

The next day, Wednesday, finally arrived and the contact with Patricia Mischell was made. She gave me some very interesting information in the phone conversation (which is also on tape). Although some things in this reading, like what Heather is doing on the other side, are unprovable, there are things in the reading that were virtually impossible for her to have known.

Some of the most outstanding information she gave me

is worth sharing here. One of the first things she told me was that Heather had fought so hard for her life. She actually used the phrase, "she fought for every breath" to stay in this realm. She asked me if I remembered how Heather had held on to me before she died. No one else in this world knew this, except me.

She next told me of the significance of the rose between Heather and me. She told me that Heather was standing in a bed of roses and extending a rose to Walt and me. She told me that a rose, no matter how I would receive it, would be a symbol of the bond between Heather and me.

She mentioned that I had visitations from Heather and asked me about these. She mentioned the importance of her coming to me in dreams. She strongly emphasized that I was intuitive and that Heather just knew that I would eventually figure this out. Patricia herself questioned me as to the meaning of this. I later explained to her that I had been in a mind-control system at the time of Heather's death and would, therefore, not be a likely candidate for this kind of experience. Patricia was surprised.

She next told me something that made a tremendous impact on me. Only the editor at A.R.E. Press and a few close friends had seen the original manuscript. Yet she suddenly stunned me when she said, "Tell Mom not to forget, it's 'Pennies from heaven.' " I actually gasped when she said this. She asked me why. When I explained to Patricia, she, too, was amazed.

She stunned me again when she told me that Heather had come as a "ball of light"! How could she be getting this? It was information that was so minute (compared to the full scope of things) that I did not have any conscious thoughts, questions, or needs regarding this. I had been more consciously focused on names, dates, and places.

Yet the more I thought about it and the more I listened to the tape, the more I could see that it is just this kind of information that makes psychic ability believable. She could not have readily accessed any of this information through ordinary means, yet some of these accounts were in the original manuscript that was now in the hands of A.R.E. Press. I was so moved.

She told me a lot of other personal things about myself, Martti, Heather, and the family that she would have no way of knowing. Everything she told me was correct. Even the circumstances surrounding Heather's death as compared to Martti's death were correct, yet known by very few people.

She closed with the fact that a single rose would be my symbol of Heather. She emphasized that Heather was present at celebrations and that I was to continue my creative project.

When I asked Patricia if the creative project she was referring to meant a book, she said it certainly could be and asked me why. When I told her about this book, she said that it would be published and that a rose would be received before the news about the book came. I hung up the phone feeling charged with energy.

Walt and I quickly changed and went to get Kim to take her out to dinner for her graduation celebration. As we entered the restaurant, we noticed that every table had a single red rose on it. We laughed and cried at the same time. There are many classy restaurants in Rhode Island. Very few use roses on every table on a Wednesday evening, especially a Wednesday two weeks before Christmas. Most restaurants had Christmas reminders on their tables. Yet we sat and even took a picture of the rose on our table. I glowed with energy as I reflected on what Patricia had told me.

The next morning, I went for my hour-long walk. As I walked along my usual route, I noticed a penny. I laughed as I said out loud, "Pennies from heaven." I stopped laughing when I got home and put my glasses on; the date of the penny was 1972. That was the year that Heather was born.

Of all the pennies I had collected, I had never found a penny that had a significant date on it. Today I would find

Heather's birth-year penny. I could feel the emotion of joy coming over me again.

Friday night we went to dinner. We had a wonderful evening. When we came out, I went to get into the car and very obviously in the middle of the floor mat was a shining penny. No one else had been in this new car yet. It was very possible that I or Walt could have dropped one, but why tonight? Why had I not noticed this penny when I got into the car? When we got home, I looked at the date, 1994. What could this mean? Time for a new beginning?

A week later, the penny thing seemed to run its gamut. Again, on my walk, I found a penny. Again, I smiled and said, "Pennies from heaven." And, again, when I got home to look at the date with my glasses—1990, the year Heather died—I had found another significant date.

To me, the series of pennies represented a symbol of Heather's birth, her death, and a door to a new beginning. Patricia herself had admonished me to go on with my life. She told me that Heather was so radiant and so happy in the other realm. Although I cannot prove this part, I believe it to be true because of the verifiable parts of the reading that she had correctly given. She never told me that I needed her services again or that I must do something to insure Heather's well-being on the other side. I needed no money to pay for her ransom, so to speak. So what did this psychic have to gain by what she told me? The provables are true; the unprovables bring me great peace.

I was no longer surprised by all of this; neither were the friends who saw the pennies. We have reached the stage of acceptance. We feel that they are signs along the way to verify that the path we are on is correct and to urge us to persevere in our journeys.

January 1995 ushered in much promise and much impatience. In my heart, I was sure that A.R.E. Press was meant to publish Heather's story because of the way it had evolved. Yet, it seemed to be taking more time than I had anticipated it would take. Perhaps, I was wrong in my assumption.

I was very restless the first Friday in January of 1995. I prayed silently all day for a sign that A.R.E. Press would accept my manuscript. Walt sensed my restlessness and offered to take me out to dinner. Of course, I eagerly accepted.

We had a lovely dinner. On the way home, Walt decided to stop and get some ice cream for the house. He walked out of Cumberland Farms with some vanilla ice cream and a red rose. I burst into tears.

He looked at me startled and asked me why I was crying. I said to him, "You have just given me my answer. A.R.E. Press will publish this story. And the answer couldn't have come from a more beautiful source, the co–creator of Heather (her Dad)."

He asked me why I thought this to be true. I told him that I had been praying for a sign all day about the book and that I had become weary since the day was about to end. Then, when he walked out of a convenience store (not a florist) at 9:00 p.m. with a rose, I felt that this was truly an answer to my prayer. The rose had answered me again.

I asked him why he bought the rose. He said that he was at the counter paying for the ice cream when he noticed the rose. He said that he instantly thought of Heather when he saw the rose, so he thought that he should buy one for me. He had no way of knowing that I was silently praying for an answer. Again, a thought, a rose, an answer?

The following Wednesday, January 11, 1995, at approximately 5:30 p.m. on the first snowy night of the winter, Ken from A.R.E. Press called to tell me the good news. They had decided that day to accept my book proposal. Wow! I was pleased for several reasons.

First, of course, was that my book was finally accepted. Second, the rose that Walt had bought me was still sitting there on my kitchen counter when the call came in. Third, it was my daughter Kim's birthday. I had been blessed once before on this date when Kim entered my world as my first born. Now, as a birthday present to her, her baby sister's story would be told.

And fourth, the snow was another sign. The previous winter, I was the driver on Wednesday for Martti's radiation treatments. Since we were bombarded with snow weekly during that season, we always wondered who would have to drive on those snow days. Wednesday was the day it inevitably picked to snow. Martti nicknamed me his "snow bunny" and told me that he was sure that it would snow every Wednesday. We both laughed at this.

As I stood talking to Ken on the phone, I was also looking out the window and watching the snow come steadily down. We had to cancel Kim's birthday celebration due to the snow—the first snow of this winter season.

Through my laughter and my tears, I rejoiced in the miracle of my Kim's birth and the birth of Heather's book. I thanked God for this privilege. I also held a reverent moment of silence for the rose which reflected Heather and for the falling snow which reflected Martti. I asked God to remember them and to hold them close in His arms.

I was truly overwhelmed on this Wednesday, January 11, 1995; a new door had just opened for me. My prayer is that it will honor the real essence of true love, an unconditional and everlasting love.

19

Philosophically Speaking

"For as he thinketh in his heart, so is he..." Proverbs 23:7

MY BLANK CANVAS was full. The dots and lines were connecting, and the picture was finally emerging. Wait. It's changing again.

I stood in awe as I realized that it was a kaleidoscope emerging, constantly changing, constantly expanding, constantly growing, never stagnant. Wow! This was truly awesome.

"That's it," I thought. We are energy in constant motion (in spirit) even while we reside in our vehicles on earth. Our spirituality can never be stagnant or too rigid. Perhaps that is the whole point of our existence on this earth. We must try to seize every moment for positive growth as we move along with this kaleidoscopic effect.

We reside today in a paradoxical world where good and evil exist side by side.

In the past whenever I would see a TV show of starving people, I would change the channel. I couldn't bear to see the pain and suffering, and I could not understand it.

Today, I still change the channel because I can't bear to see all the pain, and I still don't understand it. But I find a legitimate (and, be careful, there are some that are not) organization that works with global problems. I try to choose to be a part of the solution by donating to a possible source of aid because, in essence, good and evil can also be expressed in terms of a problem or a solution. If we don't actively seek to be a part of the solution, we inadvertently are remaining a part of the problem. We must choose.

The person I once was would have said, "Oh, what's the use? I can't fix the world." The person I am now accepts that while fixing the whole world is beyond my abilities, I can still choose to be a part of the solution rather than part of the problem.

We must care about our fellow humans enough to actively think of ways to show love. Thoughts are very powerful things indeed. I love the quote by Hadewijch of Antwerp (a thirteenth-century mystic) which says, "We must love the humanity in order to reach the divinity." Although I realize that I have very few concrete and provable answers any more, I am so grateful for having been given the freedom to think.

I had forgotten that I am more than just a physical body. I believe that many other people on this earth have forgotten this as well. We only reside in our bodies for a period of time in order to accomplish a purpose or reach a goal. Whether we choose this to happen or whether God has provided this growth for us is an important question that each one of us must discern for ourselves. Sad to say, many of us have forgotten the spirit that we really are inside, the real self. I definitely thought that I was only my vehicle.

Perhaps the biggest tragedy that occurs with this obsession with our vehicles is connected with fear and judgment. Far too often we judge people by the vehicle that they are driving.

We don't like someone because they are in a red car. Or we think we are better than someone else because we are in a blue car. It's really sort of absurd when you view it in this light.

Just consider the world of humankind for a moment. How many murders have been committed because people felt that their race, their religion, their position in life, their political structure, their culture, their education (or whatever it may be) was superior or the only way to go. Do we really believe that we are just the vehicle?

I find it very healthy and empowering to view my life in a personal relationship with a loving creator and to believe that I was created in love, to love, and to focus on the positive loving of humanity. This gives me tremendous potential to grow.

I was recently asked, since I have quoted from the Bible so often, if I were implying that the Bible was the only sacred text on the earth. My answer is, "Absolutely not!" I quote from it because I am most familiar with this particular sacred text.

There are many sacred texts on this earth. I do caution, however, that interpretation of any of these should be an individual thing. There is nothing wrong with sharing and discussing sacred text. But, from my point of view, they all have individual application depending on the person, the time in one's life, and the circumstances involved. Don't let others try to use these texts to judge you.

In spite of how much I have learned and experienced, I am still left with an unanswered question. Most religious people believe in miracles. They would, therefore, agree that God has the power to intervene in people's lives to save them if He so chooses. The Bible is full of examples of this and so are other sacred texts. So, it's logical at this point to assume that He could have saved Heather if He chose to do so. He could also end the suffering on the earth today, immediately, if He so chose.

The obvious question for me is, "Why didn't He save my Heather?" And, "Why doesn't He end the suffering?" How can I integrate this with the concept of a loving God? Surely, these are valid questions.

It's interesting to note, however, how uncomfortable many religious people get over this issue. Yet, if we consider that the Bible defines God as Love, we must somehow be able to harmonize love with the idea that evil is permitted to occur.

That is what I have attempted to do for myself during these last five years of personal experience, counseling, research, prayer, and meditation. And that is what I intend to do with the rest of the years that I have in this lifetime. My personal philosophy as expressed in this book is a very healing one for me.

I urge people to accept the challenge and to accept responsibility for themselves. We are much more than our vehicles. Don't allow others to govern your life.

Carl Jung spoke of the "collective unconscious" and the power of thoughts. So does Edgar Cayce. The medical/psychological community also gives power to thoughts. Yet, by far, the greatest advocate of this concept was Jesus Himself.

In addition, we are hearing of case after case of NDEs (near-death experiences) and past-life remembrances. We are hearing of people, like myself, who have experienced contact with those who have passed over to the other side. Why now?

Perhaps institutions have tried to limit God's personal involvement with each and every one of us. So perhaps God is showing us that there is more to Him than what many of us have been traditionally taught to believe.

Don't be as I once was: so afraid of dying that I never learned to live. Let no event, no person, nor any organization deprive you of your rightful prize. Think positively. Love positively.

Wake up, my friend. Don't be afraid. Live your life with love and dignity. Your deliverance is inevitable. God bless you on your journey.

Bibliography

Allen, Steve. *Steve Allen on the Bible, Religion, and Morality.* Buffalo, N.Y.: Prometheus Books, 1990.

Baigent, Michael, and Leigh, Richard. *The Dead Sea Scrolls Deception.* New York, N.Y.: Summit Books, 1991.

Barthel, Manfred. *What the Bible Really Says.* Avenal, N.J.: Wings Books, 1992.

Borysenko, Joan. *Fire in the Soul.* New York, N.Y.: Warner Books, Inc., 1993.

Bramblett, John. *When Goodbye Is Forever—Learning to Live Again After the Loss of a Child.* New York, N.Y.: Ballantine Books, 1991.

Brinkley, Dannion. *Saved by the Light.* New York, N.Y.: Villard Books, 1994.

Burnham, Sophy. *A Book of Angels.* New York, N.Y.: Ballantine Books, 1990.

Callanan, Maggie, and Kelley, Patricia. *Final Gifts.* New York, N.Y.: Poseidon Press, 1992.

Cayce, Hugh Lynn. *God's Other Door.* Virginia Beach, Va.: A.R.E. Press, 1958.

Cerminara, Gina. *Many Mansions—The Edgar Cayce Story on Reincarnation.* New York, N.Y.: New American Library, 1967.

Crossan, John Dominic. *The Historical Jesus.* New York, N.Y.: HarperCollins Publishers, 1991.

Eadie, Betty J. *Embraced by the Light.* Placerville, Calif.: Gold Leaf Press, 1992.

Evans-Wentz, W. Y. *The Tibetan Book of the Dead.* London, England: Oxford University Press, 1960.

Franz, Raymond. *Crisis of Conscience.* Atlanta, Ga.: Commentary Press, 1992.

Franz, Raymond. *In Search of Christian Freedom.* Atlanta, Ga.: Commentary Press, 1991.

Furst, Jeffrey. *Edgar Cayce's Story of Attitudes and Emotions.* New York, N.Y.: Berkley Books, 1976.

Gaer, Joseph. *How the Great Religions Began.* New York, N.Y.: Dodd, Mead & Company, 1956.

Howard, Jane M. *Commune with the Angels.* Virginia Beach, Va.: A.R.E. Press, 1992.

Jonsson, Carl Olof, and Herbst, Wolfgang. *The "Sign" of the Last Days—When?* Atlanta, Ga.: Commentary Press, 1987.

Komp, Diane M., M.D. *A Window to Heaven.* Grand Rapids, Michigan: Zondervan Publishing House, 1992.

Kübler-Ross, Elisabeth. *Living with Death and Dying.* New York, N.Y.: Macmillan, 1982.

Kübler-Ross, Elisabeth. *On Death and Dying.* New York, N.Y.: Macmillan, 1970.

Lamsa, George M. *Idioms in the Bible Explained and a Key to the Original Gospel.* New York, N.Y.: HarperCollins Publishers, 1985.

Lamsa, George M. *New Testament Light.* New York, N.Y.: Harper & Row, Publishers, Inc., 1968.

Mack, Burton L. *The Lost Gospel—The Book of Q.* New York, N.Y.: HarperCollins Publishers, 1993.

Macrone, Michael. *Brush Up on Your Bible!* New York, N.Y.: HarperCollins Publishers, 1993.

Maltz, Betty. *My Glimpse of Eternity.* Tarrytown, N.Y.: Fleming H. Revell Company, 1977.

Martin, Joel, and Romanski, Patricia. *Our Children Forever: George Anderson's Messages from Children on the Other Side.* New York, N.Y.: Berkley Books, 1994.

Martin, Joel, and Romanski, Patricia. *We Are Not Forgotten: George Anderson's Messages of Hope from the Other Side.* New York, N.Y.: G. P. Putnam's Sons, 1991.

Martin, Joel, and Romanski, Patricia. *We Don't Die: George Anderson's Conversations with the Other Side.* New York, N.Y.: G. P. Putnam's Sons, 1988.

McArthur, Bruce. *Your Life: Why It Is the Way It Is and What You Can Do About It.* Virginia Beach, Va.: A.R.E. Press, 1993.

Moody, Raymond A., Jr., M.D. *Coming Back.* New York, N.Y.: Bantam Books, 1991.

Moody, Raymond A., Jr., M.D. *Life After Life.* Atlanta, Ga.: Mockingbird Books, 1975.

Moody, Raymond A., Jr., M.D. *The Light Beyond.* New York, N.Y.: Bantam Books, 1988.

Moody, Raymond A., Jr., M.D. *Reflections on Life After Life.* Atlanta, Ga.: Mockingbird Books, 1977.

Morrell, David. *Fireflies.* New York, N.Y.: E. P. Dutton, 1988.

Morse, Melvin, M.D. *Closer to the Light.* New York, N.Y.: Villard Books, 1990.

Oyler, Chris. *Go Toward the Light.* New York, N.Y.: New American Library, 1988.

Pagels, Elaine. *The Gnostic Gospels.* New York, N.Y.: Random House, 1979.

Peck, M. Scott, M.D. *The Road Less Traveled.* New York, N.Y.: Simon and Schuster, 1978.

Reed, David A. *How to Rescue Your Loved Ones from the Watchtower.* Grand Rapids, Michigan: Baker Book House Company, 1989.

Ring, Kenneth. *Heading Toward Omega.* New York, N.Y.: William Morrow & Company, 1984.

Ritchie, George G., Jr., M.D. *My Life After Dying.* Norfolk, Va.: Hampton Roads Publishing Co., Inc., 1991.

Robinson, Lytle. *Edgar Cayce's Story of the Origin and Destiny of Man.* New York, N.Y.: Berkley Books, 1976.

Sarnoff Schiff, Harriet. *The Bereaved Parent.* New York, N.Y.: Crown Publishers, 1977.

Sechrist, Elsie R. *Death Does Not Part Us.* Virginia Beach, Va.: A.R.E. Press, 1992.

Siegel, Bernie S., M.D. *How to Live Between Office Visits.* New York, N.Y.: HarperCollins Publishers, 1993.

Siegel, Bernie S., M.D. *Love, Medicine, and Miracles.* New York, N.Y.: Harper & Row, Publishers, 1986.

Siegel, Bernie S., M.D. *Peace, Love, and Healing.* New York, N.Y.: Harper & Row, Publishers, 1989.

Spong, John Shelby. *The Easter Moment.* New York, N.Y.: Harper & Row, Publishers, Inc., 1980.

Spong, John Shelby. *Living in Sin.* New York, N.Y.: HarperCollins Publishers, 1988.

Spong, John Shelby. *Rescuing the Bible from Fundamentalism.* New York, N.Y.: HarperCollins Publishers, 1991.

Stearn, Jess. *Edgar Cayce—The Sleeping Prophet.* New York, N.Y.: Bantam Books, 1967.

Sugrue, Thomas. *There Is a River: The Story of Edgar Cayce.* Virginia Beach, Va.: A.R.E. Press, 1970.

Thurston, Mark. *Discovering Your Soul's Purpose.* Virginia Beach, Va.: A.R.E. Press, 1984.

Visiting Nurse Services, Hospice Department. *When Death Is Near.* Rhode Island: VNS, 11/93/500/M.

Weiss, Brian L., M.D. *Many Lives, Many Masters.* New York, N.Y.: Simon & Schuster, 1988.

Weiss, Brian L., M.D. *Through Time into Healing.* New York, N.Y.: Simon & Schuster, 1992.

Wilson, A. N. *Jesus.* New York: W.W. Norton & Company, Inc., 1992.

Woodward, Mary Ann. *Edgar Cayce's Story of Karma.* New York, N.Y.: Berkley Publishing Group, 1984.

Yogananda, Paramahansa. *Autobiography of a Yogi.* Bombay, India: Jaico Publishing House, 1946.